D1545202

Yoga After 50

by Larry Payne, Ph.D.
Cofounder, International Association of Yoga Therapists

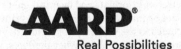

Real Possibilities

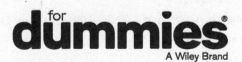

A Wiley Brand

Yoga After 50 For Dummies®

Published by: John Wiley & Sons, Inc., 111 River Street, Hoboken, NJ 07030-5774, www.wiley.com

Contents at a Glance

Table of Contents

Introduction

There is an old adage that says, "When the student is ready, the teacher will appear." For almost four decades, I've dedicated my life to being such a teacher to anyone eager to learn more about Yoga. I know firsthand that the right teacher, at the right time, can make all the difference. And I also know that Yoga can profoundly reshape your life, if you want it to.

When it comes to practicing Yoga, the key is to discover a personal approach that addresses your specific needs. Whether you use this book in addition to Yoga at your neighborhood studio, with online sessions, or on your own, I wrote Yoga After 50 for Dummies specifically to address your needs — if you happen to be over 50.

About This Book

Yoga is about so much more than postures or movements. In fact, the idea of focusing on poses is a relatively modern approach. Yoga, in fact, offers a philosophy for living and attaining joy — a philosophy for living that guides almost all aspects of our life.

Of course, postures and movements, combined with proper breathing, can have a significant impact on your health. In no way do I want to diminish both the physical and mental boost that a regular Yoga practice has to offer. Certainly, the concept of Yoga therapy is based on just that. What I am suggesting, however, is that Yoga offers a lot more than exercise.

In this book, I address the physical aspects of Yoga and beyond:

>> **Physical Yoga practice:** I spend a good portion of this book talking to you about the physical and mental benefits of Yoga, including instructions for postures, movements, and breath work. But, more precisely, I talk to you about practicing Yoga when you're over 50. I think it's critical to adjust your routines to fit your body. And it's equally important to know that such adjustments in no way diminish the fundamental concepts of Yoga practice or philosophy.

>> **Yoga beyond the poses:** How you live your life, the choices you make, can all be guided by Yoga principles. I share those ideas with you and suggest they just may be good for you, too!

As a matter of fact, Yoga in general should feel good to you and be good for you. If it doesn't, and if it leads to some kind of discomfort, you may not be recognizing what your body is telling you.

Before you listen to me or any other Yoga teacher, talk to your doctor about beginning or continuing a Yoga practice (this is especially important for all of us). And, most importantly, pay attention to how you are feeling. Nobody truly knows except you.

Foolish Assumptions

Although anyone new to Yoga or anyone who wants to practice Yoga in a more user-friendly way can benefit from this book, I'm definitely focusing my attention on a segment of the population that doesn't get enough attention in the Yoga community: people 50 and up.

As a Yoga therapist who's been working with clients for decades, I know firsthand that people benefit from simple movement and easy breathing. You don't have to do the hardest poses or the most rigorous routines to receive the health benefits from Yoga. I want you to start with what feels good for your body and your mind, and you should make that your ongoing goal as your Yoga practice evolves.

While writing this book, I assumed that you fall into one of the following categories:

>> Yoga is something you're only thinking about trying. You've heard of the numerous health benefits a regular Yoga routine can provide but are reluctant to start because you think you're not flexible enough or that maybe Yoga is something for the younger generation. Neither of these things is true, and such concerns are actually the very reason you should jump in.

>> Yoga is something that has been a part of your life for a while. But just like professional athletes discover their body changes as they age (usually, about age 40), you're also experiencing some physical changes that require you to alter your Yoga practice to still reap the benefits.

With that in mind, my objective is to show you ways that Yoga can benefit you at any age. So, if you haven't started practicing Yoga, now is a perfect time to start. If Yoga has been a part of your life for a while, you can keep practicing, even as your body changes. In both cases, I want to help.

If you want a more comprehensive view of Yoga and many of its traditional principles, you can also check out my previous book, *Yoga For Dummies* (Wiley).

Icons Used in This Book

Several icons are used throughout the margins of this book:

TIP

This icon identifies special tips that you would typically get from your Yoga teacher.

REMEMBER

You should keep in mind certain things whenever you're doing a particular pose or activity.

WARNING

Yoga should not lead to injury. Pay attention to the warnings, which are intended to keep you safe.

Beyond the Book

If you like to get your information in slightly smaller bites, be sure to check out my access-anywhere articles on the web. I take some of the most important concepts from this book and include them in these stand-alone articles that will hopefully reinforce some of my messages and also make important information even more accessible. You can find these cheat sheets online at www.dummies.com. To get this Cheat Sheet, simply go to www.dummies.com and search for "Yoga After 50 For Dummies Cheat Sheet" in the Search box.

Where to Go from Here

Keep in mind that when it comes to Yoga, there's no simple story to tell with a beginning and an end. In fact, the reason it's called a Yoga *practice* is because that is exactly what we all do . . . we practice. Although I do outline some basic principles in the first few chapters of this book that should be important to anyone, you should view this book as a guide that you can refer to again and again.

Within the chapters of this book, I have interwoven a series of general Yoga routines that, from my almost-40 years of teaching and training, I've discovered to be particularly beneficial to the 50 and over Yogi. You'll also find routines that are directed toward certain conditions common to the 50 and up crowd.

If you're already experienced in the basics, you may want to jump to one of the chapters that holds particular relevance to you — perhaps even to the routines toward the end of the book.

In any case, remember that making modifications is the key to practicing Yoga year after year. Even the greatest of Yoga masters practiced differently as they aged. And, in many cases, it's only when we practice as older adults that we discover for ourselves that Yoga is more than just another form of exercise.

1

The Age of Yoga

IN THIS CHAPTER

» Listening to your body

» Discovering the benefits of Yoga

» Reducing stress

» Choosing the right class for you

» Experiencing the magic of PNF

» Making modifications that work for you

» Practicing without injury

Chapter **1**

Yoga Over 50 Is Just Smart

Yoga is such a brilliant way to nurture both your physical, mental, and spiritual health. The only thing you may need to do is make certain modifications that will address any changing needs and keep you safe — and keep you practicing Yoga throughout your life. That's exactly what this book will help you do.

The fact is, everyone's body is different. Everyone is born with certain innate abilities, as well as certain limitations. Additionally, whether you're in your thirties or in your eighties, age may also carry with it certain limitations. All humans may be similar in structure, but each person has very specific needs.

Understanding the Benefits of Yoga

There are numerous benefits from doing Yoga. Some benefits have been scientifically measured, others have yet to be medically proven. Regardless, most everyone who tries Yoga or does Yoga regularly often talks about having a better sense of overall well-being and having more energy. Best of all, there are many aspects of Yoga you can use outside of a Yoga class. Among them are better posture and balance, improved strength and flexibility, and breathing techniques that can calm down your system in stressful situations.

A lot of Yoga offered today can be fast-paced, which may not work for you. On the other end is a chair Yoga class or Restorative Yoga. Unfortunately, there aren't a lot of classes in-between.

So, this book is part of that in-between. It shows you that you don't have to do the hardest version of a posture to receive the greatest benefits. Whether you're just beginning Yoga or you want to continue practicing Yoga throughout your life, this book identifies some of the modifications you can make that will allow you to start or to continue reaping the benefits of Yoga, including:

>> Reduced stress

>> Better sleep

>> Improved circulation

>> Improved strength and flexibility

>> Greater will power and an overall sense of well-being

As your body continues to change with age, you need to pursue a type of Yoga that adapts to those changing needs. Yet so few Yoga classes — or YouTube videos or DVDs — embrace these sorts of modifications.

WARNING

If you look around your town at the Yoga classes available to you, the majority of them will have the word *flow* in the title. This word may be your first red flag because flow classes are typically fast-moving by design.

If you're new to Yoga, it may be better to stay with introductory or level one classes.

In today's world, people often have limited time for exercise and they want a Yoga class to have a cardio component. Unfortunately, the rapid tempo of some classes sometimes means you're rushed getting in and out of poses — and you don't have enough time to consider if the pose is good for you in the first place.

The early Yoga masters taught these same kinds of flowing classes, but it's critical for you to note that they were probably teaching young boys. And, indeed, these young boys most likely had very different bodies than the one you're working with now.

It's also worth noting that these very same Yoga masters started teaching differently when they began to work with middle-aged people who were not from India. Their students' needs were different and unique, and so are yours.

Yoga at 50-plus

As a Yoga therapist and teacher, I believe that Yoga should be good for you: good for your body, mind, and spirit. Indeed, I have spent a significant part of my life trying to bring the benefits of Yoga to anyone who is interested — people like you!

You're interested enough to read this book because you've tried Yoga and liked it. Or, you suspect Yoga may have something special to offer.

The truth is, Yoga can be a great practice for anyone, offering you a multitude of benefits — if you practice the type of Yoga that's right for your body. And, what's right for your body at age 20-something is probably very different from what is right at 50-something.

At age 50 and over, Yoga may help in these essential ways:

>> Keeps muscles, bones, and joints from losing density, length, and flexibility

>> Sustains mobility with greater ease of movement

>> Protects against falling down and incurring injuries

>> Guards against skin from becoming thinner, looser, and more easily damaged

>> May help recover from some injuries faster

Yoga reduces stress

The ability of Yoga to reduce stress is widely known, and it may, in fact, be your No. 1 reason for beginning a new routine or wanting to continue your existing practice. The benefits of stress reduction can include:

>> Lower blood pressure and heart rate

>> A decrease in muscle tension

>> Better sleep (including the ability to fall asleep)

>> Prevention or management of certain medical conditions that may be related to stress (including asthma, obesity, diabetes, migraines, certain gastrointestinal issues — even Alzheimer's disease)

The fact is that reducing stress can even slow down the aging process, which may be of particular interest to the 50-plus Yogi. I talk a lot in this book about reducing or eliminating stress.

Yoga helps you breathe easier

Breathing is something you've been doing automatically since the moment you were born. But what if you changed it from something that happens without thinking to a process you guide with your conscious mind?

The first reason I talk so much in this book about breathing is that shifting the process from something you don't think about to something you do gives your mind a target on which to focus. It helps focus what I'm sure is a mind that's constantly flooded with an abundance of thoughts. And when your mind is focused on a positive activity, stress and anxiety may start to dissipate.

And this point brings up the second reason I focus on breath — and why Yoga focuses so much on breath. Timing your inhalations and exhalations with specific movements can help relax your body. Basically, as you can see throughout this book, I ask you to inhale when you open up and exhale when you fold. If you follow this approach, your diaphragm moves more freely, and your stress level can be lowered because you're breathing more easily.

Later in this book I offer some deep breathing routines that will bring these feel-good promises to life for you (see Chapter 3 for details on these routines and how breath work helps to reduce stress).

Yoga helps your body

Many of my private clients come or have come from the world of professional sports, and I was initially surprised that most of them decided to retire somewhere around the age of 40. Why? Because their bodies were changing. Yours may be, too — but Yoga can help you counter many of the typical effects of aging.

When you are of an age when you need reading glasses, that's not negotiable. But perhaps the best news about Yoga is that it can help your body mature gracefully. Yoga can counter common events such as muscles starting to feel stiff and less flexible. Every muscle in your body is subject to these changes, and what specific muscles are affected is certainly determined by how and by how much you move on a daily basis.

With a regular Yoga practice, you will most likely avoid pulling your back while bending over to make a bed or straining your back picking up something off the floor.

Movement

There's a lot of power derived from simple movement. I can certainly see this power as a Yoga teacher, and even more so as a Yoga therapist. In Yoga therapy, as I apply basic Yoga principles and techniques to help people deal with chronic conditions, I more often than not prescribe simple breath work and movement to help manage a condition or chronic pain.

In today's world, many people suffer from being too stationary. Sitting behind a desk or in front of a computer or TV may create physical or mental problems that you can often counter by easy movement.

One of my most important tenets as a Yoga teacher and therapist — and as the author of this book — is that you don't have to do the most challenging poses to reap the physical benefits.

Many of the routines in this book involve stretching your muscles. This focus on stretching will hopefully help increase both your flexibility and range of motion. These outcomes are particularly important to people 50-plus, who may be less flexible than they were years ago. More than that, inflexibility and a compromised range of motion can make you more prone to falling. The key then is to do Yoga in a safe way.

When I think of flexibility, I always think about the spine. In fact, in Yoga, spine health and mobility are my No. 1 priority. A healthy spine will keep you free from a lot of routine chronic pain, and it will improve your posture by allowing you to stand up taller and straighter.

Balance

Throughout life, learning to balance is always a challenge, but the rewards are great. As a baby, you learn to walk; as a child, you learn to ride a bike; in your teens, you may want to try a skateboard or learn to ski. Maintaining a good sense of balance is a must.

Yet balance takes practice at any age. I include in this book some Yoga poses that require balance. Don't be discouraged if you're not particularly stable at first. Your body and your brain will learn. And just like walking or riding a bike took some practice, so, too, will balance poses. Stay safe (maybe stand near a wall), and you'll get better with repetition.

Chronic conditions

So many of the chronic conditions that plague us are caused or complicated by stress and a lifestyle that keeps people sitting in front of the TV or computer and not moving enough. Those conditions include:

>> Back issues (upper and lower)

>> Breathing difficulties

>> Stress

>> Arthritis

>> High blood pressure

>> Obesity

>> Osteoporosis

>> Insomnia

>> Headaches

REMEMBER

Yoga can be a great tool in your toolbox for either preventing or managing many of these conditions by building strength and flexibility, improving the way you breathe, and reducing the amount of stress in your life. If you're just starting out or perhaps taking your existing Yoga practice to a new level, you will want to practice Yoga in a way that improves your health.

Yoga for meditation

The health benefits of meditation for anyone at any age are well documented. While some studies suggest a meditation routine can actually delay the symptoms of Alzheimer's or dementia, simply reducing your stress may have a positive impact on things like your blood pressure or those conditions associated with increased stress and anxiety. That's why I've dedicated a whole chapter to meditation in this book (see Chapter 5).

Yoga improves your mental health

I talk about how Yoga reduces stress in the section earlier in this chapter, and I make references to stress reduction throughout the book. I also focus on the link between the mind and the body and how having a healthy emotional self may also help you maintain a healthy physical self.

In Yoga, whether you're doing movements, postures, or breath work, the goal is always to steady the mind, slow your breathing and heart rate, and provide a refuge of sorts where you can find some peace and tranquility. In fact, many Yoga practitioners report better mental attitudes and better sleep, according to a study, "The Use of Yoga for Physical and Mental Health Among Older Adults: A Review of the Literature," published by the International Association of Yoga Therapists.

Check with your healthcare provider before you start

Make sure you talk to your doctor before you start a Yoga practice. I would never want to circumvent anything another healthcare provider is telling you, so don't make the decision to try Yoga without your doctor's knowledge and consent. And if you're currently not seeing a doctor, but are dealing with acute pain, jumping into Yoga is not the answer.

Finding Your Place in the World of Yoga

The challenge in putting together this book, as well as teaching any public class, is that people come to Yoga with varying degrees of experience and unique bodies. My goal is to be helpful to everyone.

If you're new to Yoga, start slowly and gently — and, most of all, be patient. Some poses will get easier with practice, and some will not. In the end, everyone is assigned a certain body type with certain abilities and limitations. In starting a new practice, you'll discover both if you pay attention.

TIP

Modifications are the key to a lifelong practice. As our bodies change, all you need to do is modify where necessary, and you'll be a practicing Yogi for the rest of your life.

You may find it very helpful to ignore your ego and compulsion to compete (even with yourself!). Forget about what you used to be able to do! It is critical to remember that Yoga needs to make you healthier, and you need to make choices that are smart for your body as it is today.

Selecting the Right Place and the Right Teacher for You

When it comes to practicing Yoga, I know you have a lot of choices. There's definitely an abundance of classes available to you, whether it's visiting a local Yoga studio or viewing a DVD or video on your computer or smartphone. The most important thing is to choose a level of instruction that is appropriate to your current level of practice. If you happen to select a class — whether it's at a studio or on a video at home — that's too advanced or even too easy, you could easily get the wrong impression about what Yoga has to offer.

Let me give you my thoughts about the various options available to you.

Selecting classes wisely

Depending on where you live, you may find Yoga studios on every other block. If so, you need to be selective.

Keep in mind that many of the flow classes or power Yoga classes are designed for people in their 20s who are looking for a more athletic experience — one that has an intense cardio component. The reality is that in today's world, people have only a limited amount of time for fitness, so — even in Yoga classes — they are looking for a session that combines stretching and strength with routines that will get their heart rate up at the same time. Unfortunately, these classes may not work for you.

WHAT IS YOGA THERAPY?

The International Association of Yoga Therapists (IAYT) defines *Yoga therapy* as "the process of empowering individuals to progress toward improved health and well-being through the application of the teachings and practices of Yoga." While a Yoga therapy session is usually conducted one-on-one (so the therapist can focus on the specific needs of the client), Yoga therapy group classes are becoming more common. In these types of classes, all the students share the same condition (maybe it's a class for people with arthritis) or the class targets a specific area of the body with the objective of maintaining health (for example, a healthy lower-back class). In all cases, whether in a one-on-one session or a group class, Yoga therapy is not intended to be a substitute for medical treatment, nor is it for people in acute pain.

Although you may see Yoga therapy-type classes that can address the specific needs of a particular population (for example, people looking for an emphasis on lower-back health), if you're dealing with a personal health issue, you should seek individualized Yoga therapy.

Again, it's not about being less motivated; it's about being smart. You don't want to be in a class where the poses or the tempo require you to practice in a way that compromises your safety. You're there to get healthy, not injured. And, as I always say, "Yoga is not in a hurry" (or at least it shouldn't be).

Choose your studios — and your classes — carefully.

TIP

Although you may see Yoga therapy-type classes that can address the specific needs of a particular population (for example, people looking for an emphasis on lower-back health), if you're dealing with a personal health issue, you should seek individualized Yoga therapy.

Of course, even general Yoga classes are ideal when they're one-on-one because the Yoga teacher can adapt the instruction to the very specific needs of the student. Private Yoga lessons, however, are a bit costly for most people.

Yoga has become so pervasive today that your choices on where to practice and whom to select as a teacher can seem infinite and definitely confusing. You can turn to a number of places where you'll find a comfortable setting and an encouraging and well-qualified teacher. The critical first step is to make a thoughtful choice.

Although no one place or teacher is right for everyone, you need both to be right for you. If you're a novice and you find yourself in a class that's designed for more experienced Yogis, or if you discover your teacher is too aloof or perhaps lacking in knowledge, please move onto another option so you don't miss out on the many benefits Yoga can offer you.

YOGA TRENDS

It has been exciting to see ancient Yoga practices evolve into so many branches to serve modern needs. *For example, some styles of Yoga fit the person to the Yoga Pose.* My style fits the Yoga positions to the person.

In any case, new forms of Yoga are always popping up, as well as Yoga hybrids: paddleboard yoga, aerial yoga, acro yoga (acrobatics and yoga), Pi-Yo Yoga (Pilates and Yoga)—even Laughing Yoga (see Chapter 7).

My concern is that many of these classes are very athletic or very rapid in tempo and not necessarily safe for everyone. The demand for these types of classes comes from the fact the most people have only a limited amount of time to work out. So, in addition to building strength and flexibility, they also want a good cardio workout — they want to burn calories. As a result, many of these newer Yoga classes do just that, but they may not be a good or a safe choice for you.

Home

In addition to the wide range of in-person classes that may be available to you in your neighborhood, you've undoubtedly come across hundreds — maybe even thousands — of Yoga DVDs to purchase or free Yoga videos on YouTube or on some other streaming services.

While many talented teachers and well-designed videos are at your disposal, your particular challenge is to find the ones that are just right for you — videos that will actually improve your health and fitness and not lead to injury. There are some great DVDs and videos out there; you need to choose carefully — and choose wisely.

Many of the videos that I've come across are designed for what I call the young and restless. If you combine an inappropriately aggressive practice with the fact that you're in front of your computer or TV instead of in the actual company of an experienced teacher who is trying to keep you safe, you may be courting injury.

Even in my own DVD series, I know that some people may have conditions that make certain postures or movements difficult or unwise. Nonetheless, I make every effort to provide the viewer with as much information as I can relating to the benefits or risks of a certain poses. In fact, the first priority of all my videos is practicing in a way that increases the benefits and minimizes the risks.

TIP

I don't want to recommend any specific video or teacher (besides this book, of course), but I do want to set the bar high. If you do try a DVD or video, you may want to look for something that is specifically designed for your age group. You may be able to determine this directly from the title. Also, look at the qualifications of the teacher. Ideally, that person will have some degree of expertise in adapting Yoga to the 50-plus body.

Gym

Some very talented teachers, as well as some great classes, are at gyms. Again, just make sure the class offers the right approach for you.

People who come to the gym tend to have only a limited amount of time to dedicate to fitness. As a result, gyms may design their classes to provide a rigorous overall workout. People who come to these classes are often looking for a cardio component, so the Yoga classes tend to be *flow classes,* which keep you moving rapidly, or *power Yoga classes,* which emphasize strength and endurance.

If you're trying a class at the gym, talk to the teacher beforehand to make sure it's the right class for you.

Houses of worship, community centers, and libraries

You can find some great classes and teachers in houses of worship, community centers, and libraries. Make sure the teacher is experienced and skilled, providing modifications for bodies of different abilities. And make sure the makeshift studio offers the right space and right props, or it's no bargain at all.

You may find that the Yoga teacher is just renting space at any of these venues.

REMEMBER

The bottom line is be selective. Make sure the type of class is appropriate for your skill level and that the teacher is good at keeping a roomful of people safe and informed.

Practicing without Injury

As the number of people attending Yoga classes continues to climb, so, too, are the number of people going to emergency rooms because they got hurt in a Yoga class. I don't want you to be one of them — and that's one of the reasons I wrote this book.

You're probably completely on board with the goals of strengthening your body, increasing your flexibility and balance, reducing stress, and breathing more mindfully. But you'll want to add one more: avoiding injury. A key problem, from my observation, is that too many people don't listen to their bodies and trust their own instincts on what postures are beneficial and which ones are risky, or heed their pain signals. Instead, they make the mistake of listening to their egos.

Sometimes, people want to keep up with their hyper-mobile, 20-something teacher, or they want to show the people practicing next to them that they are just as flexible and just as advanced, or they want to do the moves they did when they last did Yoga 20 years ago. And that is just plain foolish.

WARNING

I strongly advise you to ignore how you look in a Yoga pose, and certainly please do not compare yourself to how anyone else looks doing Yoga.

They say with age comes wisdom, and my hope is that we all bring some of that hard-won wisdom to the Yoga mat. Listen to your body; listen to your intuition; and be smarter. If you're able to do this, you will discover how Yoga can make you better, even healthier, than you are today. And there's a good chance you'll avoid injury.

Playing It Safe

As previously mentioned, preparing your muscles and joints before moving in and out of various poses helps to reduce the possibility of injury, especially from over-stretching.

Moving in and out of a pose before holding it is referred to as the dynamic/static approach which can also yield the benefits of PNF (explained in detail below).

So, then, there are a few reasons to move first before holding a pose: Mainly it lubricates your joints and helps you stretch further.

You should not only come to expect this form of movement, but I'll bet you will learn to enjoy it!

Warming up

How often do you see athletes warming up before a game or runners stretching out before breaking into a sprint? It probably makes perfect sense to you. Before moving or stressing the body in a new way, warming up seems logical.

In Yoga classes, you frequently start with a short warm-up sequence. A good teacher will always structure the class so that one posture or movement prepares the body for what's coming next.

Our bodies benefit from preparing joints and muscles before each new posture. That is why I frequently move my students in and out of poses before I ask them to hold steady. You should consider this approach as well.

One of the reasons Yoga is such an effective routine for nurturing your body is that it tries to bring movement — often stretching, sometimes strengthening — to all areas of the body. That means, at some point in your practice, whether you're in a class or by yourself at home, most all of your muscles and moveable joints will be worked.

As far as your joints go, your goal is to warm them up in such a way that focuses on specific movements (or ranges of motion). Just to be clear, your moveable joints include:

>> Ankles

>> Knees

» Hips

» Spine

» Neck

» Shoulders

» Elbows

» Wrists

I include a great routine for joint health in Chapter 16. You may want to check it out.

Of course, if you have any joint replacements, you need to consider a few additional items. For that, please refer to Chapter 14.

Preparing the joints

If joints like your knees and ankles are designed to move, the joints themselves must be properly lubricated. Just like in your car, proper lubrication reduces the amount of friction between moving parts.

Moving in and out of a pose before holding it helps to distribute the lubrication (called *synovial fluid*) to all parts of the joint.

Take, for example, a simple hip rotation (see Figure 1-1). This movement is intended to focus on the hip joint — that big ball and socket where the top of your leg (your femur) fits into your hip socket. By rotating your knee in big circles, the joint is working in its full range of motion, distributing lubrication, and better preparing you for the movements to come.

No wonder football players do this exact same warm-up before taking the field for a game.

Performing magic with PNF

Another potential benefit of moving in and out of a posture is related to the concept of Proprioceptive Neuromuscular Facilitation, or PNF, that I talked about before. This topic is somewhat complex, and fitness experts debate how PNF actually prepares the muscles and joints. Nevertheless, one of the most basic aspects of PNF is this: If you tense a muscle before you try to stretch it, it will relax more.

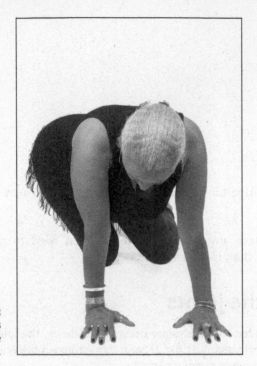

FIGURE 1-1:
Hip circles
prepare the
hip joints.

Typically, you can tense a muscle in two ways:

» **Isometric:** Pushing against a fixed force

» **Isotonic:** Tightening a muscle using gentle resistance

Isometric stretching in Yoga usually involves a partner. For example, you can lie on the floor, with a straight leg lifted up and propped against your partner (see Figure 1-2). By first pressing the heel of the lifted leg against your partner, the muscles in your leg will tighten. After holding that press for approximately eight seconds, you can release the pressure and move the leg in the opposite direction. As a result of first tensing the muscles, they will now relax further than they would have had you not tightened them first.

Of course, most of the time when you practice, no one is around to help you. This is where the dynamic/static approach comes in — moving in and out of a posture before holding it.

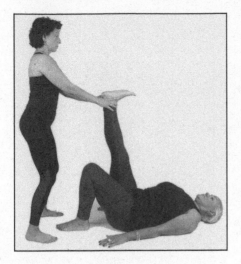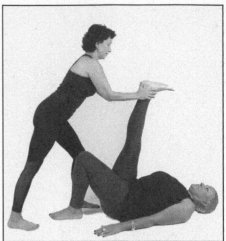

FIGURE 1-2:
PNF with
isometric
resistance.

If you perform the same movement (see Figure 1-3) by lifting and lowering your leg yourself before holding the stretch, you're actually tensing your muscles; each time you lower your leg, if you don't tense your muscles, your leg would come crashing to the ground with the force of gravity.

TIP

My rationale, then, is simple: If the PNF concept that tensing a muscle before you stretch it will ultimately allow it to stretch further, then moving in and out of a posture, before holding, may offer some of the same benefit.

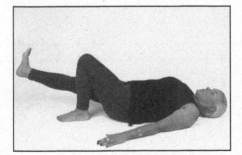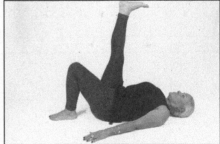

FIGURE 1-3:
PNF using
isotonic
resistance.

Modifications

Knowing your own body and what it can do on any given day is essential. Teachers should be offering and demonstrating a variety of modifications of poses. In addition, the chapters in this book provide you with some important tips and guidance for modifying Yoga to fit your particular needs.

Chapter **2**

Preparing to Practice

I t seems that, for some people, the prospect of adding Yoga to their daily or weekly routine is a bit intimidating. This chapter focuses on two of the reasons people use to avoid Yoga: I don't know what clothes to wear and I don't know what equipment to get.

The truth is, the clothes, mats, and props you choose should only serve to make your Yoga routines safer and more effective. In this chapter, my goal is to take away some of the mystery as you get ready to practice.

You Don't Need a Lot of Equipment to Practice Yoga

Unlike other physical activities, such as golf or scuba diving, you don't need a lot of expensive equipment to practice Yoga. A few items are useful to have, while some other things are completely unnecessary.

The following sections take a look at a few key items:

» Comfortable clothes

» Mats

» Blocks

>> Blankets

>> Bolsters

>> Straps and other accessories

Comfortable clothes

Yoga clothes may seem like a trivial topic to some, but some people feel like they need to spend a fortune on brand-name Yoga clothing to be accepted into the Yoga community. This assumption is decidedly not true. I spend a lot of time in this book telling you that "it's not about the pose." Now, I want to make perfectly clear that it's also "not about the clothes."

You can find various name brands of Yoga clothing. (I certainly own enough myself.) For the most part, the workmanship is great, and the clothing lasts a long time. Still, many people at all levels choose other clothing so long as it's comfortable. You don't need brand-name clothes to get good quality.

REMEMBER

The only thing your clothing needs to do is make you comfortable and allow you to bend and stretch. Anyone who makes judgments based on what people wear on the mat — or, for that matter, even how flexible they may be — is completely missing the point of Yoga in the first place. (That goes for self-judgment as well.)

WARNING

On this topic, I will mention that it is considerate to choose Yoga clothing that doesn't bring a blush to the cheek of the teacher or fellow students. I mention this point only because, from time to time, someone comes to class wearing something that is not intended to be worn in inverted poses — and no one wants an impromptu anatomy class!

WARNING

Let me say a word or two about wearing socks. I know sometimes people leave their socks on in a Yoga class because their feet get cold. But socks can be a real disadvantage, particularly in standing poses. If socks are slippery, it can make holding an already challenging posture even more difficult. Bare feet in Yoga is more than just a tradition.

Doing Yoga in bare feet is

>> Less slippery when moving in and out of poses (depending on your socks)

>> More stable for balancing poses (students often say that contacting the floor with their bare feet gives them a greater sense of stability)

>> More accommodating to muscles and ligaments as you move from posture to posture (stretch and strengthen)

There are nonslip Yoga socks on the market. Some socks even have the toes exposed. While these socks are certainly safer, I'd still consider them a compromise.

TIP

If you wear orthotics — which can be particularly helpful during the standing portion of the class — you may want to leave your socks on during class and just slip your orthotics inside your socks. You'll definitely want to use nonslip socks, but this could be a way to wear your orthotics during a Yoga class.

Mats

Technically speaking, you don't have to use a mat to practice Yoga. However, the investment has become so minimal (depending on the construction of the mat) and the benefits so numerous, I would highly recommend you get one.

Where you practice will determine how much padding you need — particularly because you'll be required to lie down or kneel down. If you're doing Yoga on a carpeted, padded floor, the thickness of your mat is probably not as important. If, however, you're practicing on a hardwood floor — or worse, even some kind of stone tile — a thicker mat is sure to provide more comfort.

A mat can also provide you with a nonslip surface on which to build your Yoga poses. Keep in mind, however, that mats can also be slippery, so take this into account as you consider price and construction. Yoga mats can range from $10 to $50, depending on the thickness and design; some are bundled with props such as a block and strap.

Your process of selecting a mat should take into account the following potential benefits:

» **Personal comfort:** A mat can be especially important on a hard floor.

» **Designated space:** A mat establishes your own space (which may be particularly important in a group class).

» **More stability:** A mat can provide you with a nonslip surface, particularly useful in more precarious poses. Some mats can be better than others for this purpose; find out whether your mat has what is called a *sticky* surface, which is designed to help keep you from slipping.

Blocks

Blocks can be very useful props, allowing you to go more deeply into a posture than you would be able to do on your own. They're often used to help you reach the floor, sometimes allowing your body to reap the benefits of a particular pose. (See Figures 2-1 and 2-2.) Years ago, most blocks were made of wood; now they are lighter, often made of Styrofoam. Although they come in all different sizes, the average block measures about 9 x 6 x 4 inches.

TIP

The first thing a block can do is bring the floor closer to you so that you can perform the most beneficial aspect of the pose. Let me give you an example using triangle pose.

Notice in Figure 2-1 that the model is touching the floor with her right hand, which, in turn, causes her left shoulder to rotate inward and downward.

In Figure 2-2, however, she uses a block to bring the floor closer to her and, as a result, is able to fully open her left shoulder, reaping the full benefits of the pose. Even with the block, this execution is definitely more advanced than in the previous photograph.

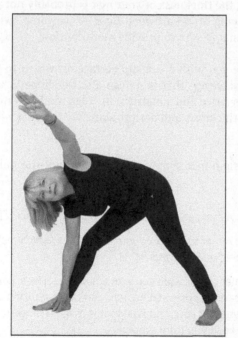

FIGURE 2-1:
Triangle pose with no block.

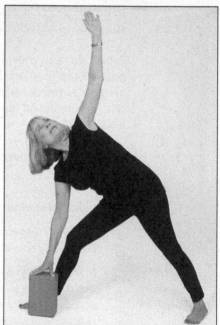

FIGURE 2-2:
Triangle pose with a block.

Of course, you can modify the pose in other ways and still get the benefits. But if a block is available, you may want to consider how it can help you get more out of a particular pose.

You will also want to consider the block construction. The most common types are:

>> Foam

>> Cork

>> Wood

Foam blocks are great for either lifting your hips, such as in a supported shoulder stand, or squeezing between your thighs to activate your inner-thigh muscles.

You can also use blocks for support or stability (again, look at Figure 2-2, where the block also provides support as she leans sideways). For support, you may prefer a block made of a firmer material.

Blankets

A good Yoga blanket can be an essential tool. It potentially offers a

>> Cushion for your head when reclining

>> Cushion for your knees when kneeling or on all fours

>> Lift for your spine, with some added comfort, when sitting

>> Cushion for your pelvis (or even face) when lying on your stomach (prone)

Like most accessories discussed in this chapter, the quality of the material can be a factor. If it is too thin, it will be hard to fold it up enough to find true comfort. And it also needs to stand up to regular washing.

I often recommend a blanket when employing some kind of modification. For example, even in easy pose, a simple seated position, a blanket under the hips helps to make the spine straighter without being forced to engage certain muscles (see Figure 2-3). You sit taller, and it's easier on your back.

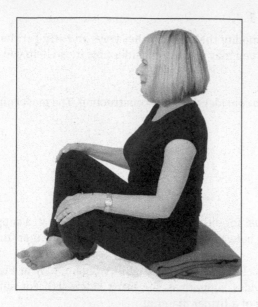

FIGURE 2-3:
Easy pose with
a blanket.

I also use blankets a lot when I see someone who is lying down and their chin is tilted way back. A blanket is a great way to cushion the head and get the chin back to a normal position (see Figure 2-4).

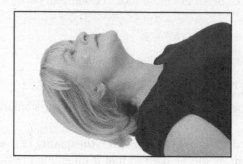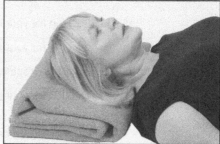

FIGURE 2-4:
Blankets helps a
tilted chin.

Bolsters, cushions, and pillows

Bolsters are designed to provide you with comfort and support in various Yoga poses. You do see bolsters used a lot in Restorative Yoga, in which you mostly stay seated or flat on the floor on your back. This type of Yoga focuses less on movement and more on breath in comfortable positions.

A *Yoga bolster* is essentially a cushion intended to provide you with additional comfort. Take child's pose, for example. If you think it's comfortable without using a bolster (or maybe you don't), try it with one (see Figure 2-5).

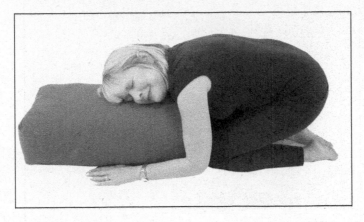

FIGURE 2-5:
Child's pose with
a bolster.

While some Yoga studios may have bolsters on hand, you probably don't have one lying around the house. No worries. You can use a folded-up blanket or even a couch or bed cushion.

In any case, a bolster or pillow may be the perfect solution when you want something soft underneath you.

Straps and other accessories

Straps are quite common in a lot of classes. You can use straps to stretch your hips and hamstring, or to constrain your arms in certain poses that tend to make your elbows want to splay open. I wouldn't use one, though, unless you're being instructed by a teacher.

I also want to mention wedges. Because wrist problems seem more common in a 50-and-up population, a wedge can be a nice way to decrease the bending angle on certain poses. They are a relatively inexpensive prop and may be quite useful.

A wedge works especially well when you're on your hands and knees (see Figure 2-6).

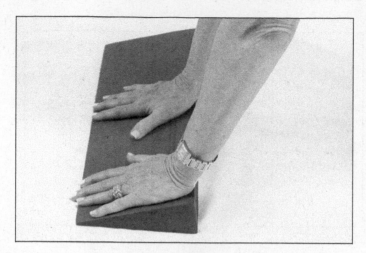

FIGURE 2-6:
Using a wedge.

Of course, if you have wrist issues, you can skip certain poses altogether — or perhaps try making fists with your hands instead of flexing your wrists (see Figure 2-7).

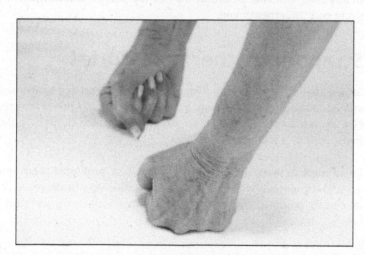

FIGURE 2-7:
Making fists.

You can check out all the other types of Yoga accessories available to you and see what might be useful. While most of my routines are designed so that you don't need props of any kind, I would encourage you to acquire anything that will make it more likely for you to get on the mat and move.

Proper Sequencing

While determining the best sequence for a Yoga routine may only be the purview of Yoga teachers, I want to talk about it here because I know you'll be tempted to look at the various Yoga postures depicted in this book and create your own routine. While that's okay, be sure to give a great deal of consideration when creating any Yoga sequence.

You can use several approaches to sequence your practice or a class. For example, a sequence may lead up to what is called a *peak pose*. Or you may focus on a particular type of pose, such as hip-openers or twists.

As usual, I don't want to champion a particular approach, but rather talk a little bit about my primary focus when creating the routines in this book.

My focus when creating a sequence of movements and postures is

>> Can I prepare your body for what's to come?

>> Can I compensate your body for something you just did?

For example, in a particular sequence, I may choose a pose or movement designed to work the abdominal muscles — say, some kind of Yoga crunches (see Figure 2-8).

In a crunch, every time the student raises her head and chest, she is shortening (or contracting) her abdominal muscles. Repeating these contractions over and over again is what helps to build strength.

Following these contractions, however, I have the opportunity to compensate for this movment. By putting the student into a bridge pose (see Figure 2-9), those very same abdominals muscles are now being lengthened and relaxed.

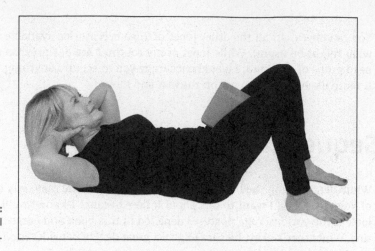

FIGURE 2-8:
Yoga abdominal
crunches.

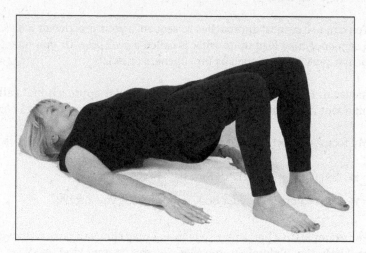

FIGURE 2-9:
Bridge pose.

Not only does this bridge pose provide some compensation for the previous abdominal work, but take a look at Figure 2-9 to see how I am stretching the muscles around the neck and shoulders. The bridge pose is also preparing the neck for going into a supported half shoulder stand pose. So, the bridge pose is actually compensating for the crunches and preparing the body for the upcoming inversion (see Figure 2-10).

While it may be unrealistic to think that every pose compensates for something that just happened or prepares for something to come (or both), every good Yoga sequence is constructed with that thought in mind, in a logical way.

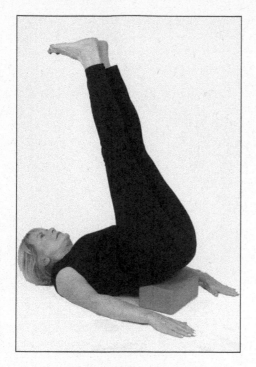

FIGURE 2-10:
Supported
shoulder stand.

Before You Begin

Before you begin, gather the following items:

>> Clothing that's comfortable and will let you move

>> A mat (thick enough to accommodate the flooring)

>> A blanket (to lift your spine, cushion your knees, or even just keep you warm)

>> A towel (in case you get sweaty)

>> Water (to help you stay hydrated)

WARNING

Be sure it is okay with your doctor or other healthcare provider that you are going to practice Yoga.

Chapter **3**

Breathing through Your Yoga Poses

ow many times have you heard the expression "take a breath"? Maybe your mother gave you that instruction when she wanted you to calm down before taking an impulsive action or making a hasty decision. Perhaps you say it to yourself now before reacting too fast to an inflammatory situation.

Even outside the Yoga world, breathing and composure have a close relationship. Somehow a simple breath can decrease your level of stress and bring balance and self-control to a tense encounter or an emotional moment.

What makes Yoga unique is that it sees the breath as a fundamental part of Yoga practice and philosophy. It can be one of your most powerful tools.

You'll find more breathing exercises in Chapter 11.

Benefiting from Breathing in Yoga

As a Yoga therapist, I see firsthand the benefits of breathing exercises:

>> Reduced pain

>> Reduced blood pressure

>> Slower pulse

>> Increased relaxation

You can achieve these outcomes just by paying attention to how you're breathing and starting to take control of the process.

Leveraging Your Breathing

The thing about breathing is you've been doing it for a very long time, without thinking about it much. You have been breathing since birth, so your initial instinct may be that you certainly don't need to learn how to breathe.

REMEMBER

If you're going to leverage your breath as a tool, you don't need to learn how to breathe; you need to learn how to control your breath. Before I continue, let me make two critical points:

>> Because you've been breathing successfully your entire life, I am not going to tell you now that your breathing is wrong or right. Yoga breathing exercises are about learning to control, to take charge of, the process. One way to do so is to practice different ways to breathe.

>> One of the overall goals of Yoga is to achieve a state of calmness or peace — a steadiness of mind. You will not be working toward this goal if your breath work causes you anxiety. Don't try more difficult breathing exercises unless you are eager to learn and inspired by the challenge. You may have the option of working with a teacher, which can be a more effective way to learn the more advanced techniques.

Breathing through the nose

The first thing to consider when you're thinking about your breath is the old Yoga adage that says, "The mouth is for eating and the nose is for breathing." Inhaling and exhaling only through the nose definitely has some advantages — but only if you're able to do so comfortably.

If you happen to have a cold, allergies, or some kind of obstruction (like a deviated septum), don't try to force anything. It's not a good time to breathe through your nose alone. There are a few practical benefits of breathing through the nose, if you can. You employ the natural air filtration system that your body provides via nose hairs and the mucous lining. Also, taking in air through the nose provides temperature regulation. You can warm the air more efficiently, which is better for your lungs in any season.

While nasal breathing may have many other purported benefits, the simple fact is that the nasal passages are much smaller channels for the air to flow through than is your open mouth. As a result, you tend to breathe deeper and more slowly.

And slowing the breath — especially the exhalation — is the key.

Extending the exhalation

Even the most ancient Yoga texts talk about how powerful it is to extend your exhalation — or letting air out slowly — which can be a confusing concept. How can you expend more air than you take in?

You can't. But what you can do is lengthen your exhalation by expelling air more slowly than you took it in. If you're a singer, it's how you sing a long note; the same thing goes if you play a wind instrument.

Some of the benefits of learning to extend your exhale are first recognized in what's generally considered to be Yoga's foundational work, *The Yoga Sūtras of Patañjali* (Simon & Schuster) translated by Georg Feuerstein. In fact, Sutra 1.34, dedicated entirely to this subject, says that one way to quiet the mind and maximize joy is to extend the exhale: "[Y]ou can try lengthening the exhale and observe the pauses in between breaths to cultivate a calm and clear mind."

More recently, Tim McCall, M.D., explains, "Lengthening exhalation relative to inhalation reduces the 'fight or flight' impulse and maintains a healthy level of carbon dioxide in the blood, which helps you relax." You can see his complete discussion in the *Yoga Journal* at www.yogajournal.com/practice/buzz-away-the-buzzing-mind.

If you're not familiar with slowing down your exhalation, some of the breathing exercises in this chapter can help you practice just that.

Extending your exhalation ultimately sends a text-like message to your brain, often resulting in:

>> Slower heart rate

>> Lower blood pressure

>> Relaxed muscles and mind

>> Better digestion

This message stimulates your parasympathetic nervous system and says you are safe. As a result, your brain doesn't need to help you by producing the stress hormones (like adrenaline or cortisol) you would need if you planned on running away or staying and fighting. Instead, you relax.

Four-part breathing

It is customary to think of your breath as being in two parts: the inhalation and the exhalation. But, if you think about it, you really breathe in four parts:

>> Inhalation

>> Slight pause

>> Exhalation

>> Slight pause

To practice the four-part breath, your Yoga instructor may ask you to increase the time it takes to inhale and exhale, and even increase the pauses. But if you're not accustomed to this type of breath work, the breathing may actually increase your level of anxiety.

I'm suggesting instead that you focus on the four-part aspect of your breathing — and that will be enough. In fact, it may also be easier to keep your mind focused if you're concentrating on a breathing pattern that you're not used to doing.

Breath surrounds movement

Yoga philosophy stresses the relationship between the breath and movement. In fact, one translation for the Sanskrit word Yoga is *union*, referring to the union between breath and movement.

It is important to keep in mind the following principles when Yoga teachers instruct you to inhale or exhale as you move in and out of postures:

>> Breathe through the nose only (if possible), mouth closed, lips slightly parted.

>> Extend (lengthen) your exhale.

You'll also want to practice four-part breathing.

Generally speaking, in Yoga, the objective is very straightforward: Keep breathing slowly, no matter what pose you're doing.

WARNING

Holding your breath or breathing rapidly sends a different message to the brain. If trying to do a particular pose leads to this type of breathing, you should consider doing a less challenging (modified) version — at least until you are ready to do the pose with your breath under control.

The link between body, breath, and mind is essential. Without that link, Yoga would just be another form of exercise. Yoga is unique because it brings breath, movement, and meditation together to bring the body into stillness.

TIP

It is definitely easier to inhale in certain positions and exhale in others. That is why it is important not only to keep breathing as you move, but to breathe in a way that works well with your physical posture. In Yoga, you would typically take air in (inhale) when you open your body and extend (for example, raising your arms overhead). When you're closing your posture, you typically exhale (staying with my example, when you lower your arms back down). Coordinating your movement with your breath will help to ensure that your physical movements are compatible with your breathing process.

Three Ways to Breathe When Moving

If breath is truly going to surround your movements in Yoga, it is worth paying attention to precisely how you're breathing. I recommend taking one of the following three approaches:

>> **Focus breathing:** Breathe through the nose only. I talk about the advantages of breathing only through your nose (inhalations and exhalations) in the section earlier in this chapter. This technique is probably the easiest and a good place to start. I call this Focus breathing.

>> **Belly breathing:** Breathe through the nose only and gently pull the belly in on the exhalation. In this approach, paying attention to the rising and falling of your stomach will ensure your diaphragm is moving properly, which in turn provides stimulation to the surrounding areas, including the low back and pelvic floor. This approach is also a great way to help you relax.

>> **Chest-to-belly:** Breathe through the nose only and inhale first with your chest and then your belly. Focusing your inhalation into your chest causes your rib cage to expand and, when it does, your shoulders will open. This opening or expansion counters the effects of everyday rounding (a phenomenon that increases with age and definitely impacts the posture).

Advanced Breath Work

Breath work is an essential part of the Yoga tradition. I've even spoken to a number of experts who say that the real purpose of postures and movement in Yoga is simply to prepare the body to sit and breathe for extended periods of time. I know from my own experience that the breath can be a very powerful tool in stress and pain management.

When writing this book, I contacted an old friend in India, Ananda Balayogi Bhavanani, and asked his opinion of the best breathing routines for the 50-plus population. (Bhavanani is a medical doctor, earned a doctorate, and is a Yoga therapist.) We base our recommendations on two criteria:

>> Each routine is safe to do without a teacher present.

>> Each routine is designed to put no or minimal stress on the body.

While they're certainly not the only breath routines available to you, here are our recommendations:

>> Bellows variation

>> Left nostril breathing

>> Alternate nostril breathing

>> Bee breath

WARNING

Don't underestimate the power of your breath! Even now, without doing any exercises, you experience the positive physical sensations of a yawn or a simple sigh. In the following exercises, you explore the ways you can use your breath to re-create these same benefits — at will.

Preparing for breath work

Unlike the breathing that surrounds your movements and postures, the following exercises focus on your breathing alone. They're typically done in a comfortable seated position, which is great news because you can do them in an office or at the kitchen table.

WARNING

Please note that these breathing exercises are not meant to be a substitute for a medical diagnosis or treatment. Moreover, if performing any part of these routines causes you to start feeling dizzy or lightheaded, you may want to lie down on your back, with your eyes closed, or, if you're standing, you may want to lower to a squat and drop your chin. The bottom line is to not push through it. Give your body a chance to find its equilibrium.

To prepare the lungs for the following routines:

1. **Sit in a place that is comfortable (see Figure 3-1).**

2. **Inhale and exhale only through the nose.**

TIP

   If you can, slow down your exhalation and make it take longer than your inhalation.

3. **Continue for eight to ten breaths.**

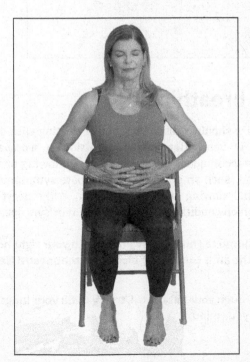

FIGURE 3-1:
Sitting posture for breath work.

Bellows variation routine

This breathing exercise is one of the few times I ask you to use your mouth. It's a relatively easy technique to perform and very effective in extending your exhalation and slowing down your breath.

1. Inhale fully through your nose only.

2. Exhale through your mouth only, making the "shhh" sound as you slowly release air (see Figure 3-2).

3. Repeat nine more times.

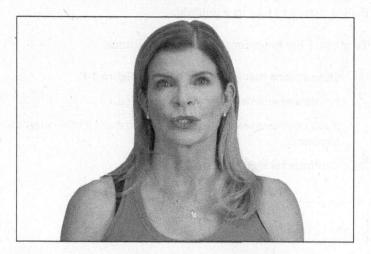

FIGURE 3-2:
Bellows variation.

Left nostril breathing

WARNING

This breathing exercise should be avoided if you're dealing with depression, your metabolism is slow, or you suffer from hypotension or *syncope* (the tendency toward fainting). The technique is intended to have a slowing or relaxing impact on the body and mind. Such an effect may exacerbate symptoms of depression. Similarly, the potential slowing of the metabolism — the heart rate and blood pressure — could worsen conditions like hypotension or syncope.

1. Use your right thumb to gently apply pressure to your right nostril, just enough so that the air is completely blocked in that nostril (see Figure 3-3).

2. Slowly inhale through your left nostril, trying to fill your lungs as you count to four in your mind.

3. Exhale through your left nostril, this time trying to slow the mental count to six or more.

4. Repeat this cycle for a total of eight more rounds, keeping your right nostril blocked the whole time.

Each time you inhale, feel yourself relaxing as you fill your lungs. As you exhale, feel your stress exiting.

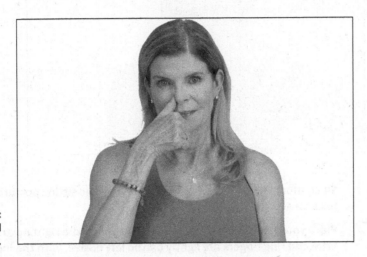

FIGURE 3-3: Left nostril breathing.

Alternate nostril breathing

Alternate nostril breathing is a great exercise to help you link your mind with your breath. You breathe through one nostril at a time instead of two. It takes a bit of concentration, but you ultimately reduce your stress level by allowing your thoughts to focus on the technique itself, and by slowing your breath rate down. Benefits include:

» Better mental balance

» Improved focus

» Reduced stress and anxiety

You have multiple options for how you want to position yourself, but sitting upright, in a comfortable chair, will probably help with your concentration if you've never done this exercise.

Use an easy hand position, making the Hawaiian hang-loose sign (see Figure 3-4) and then adding the ring finger. Then follow these steps:

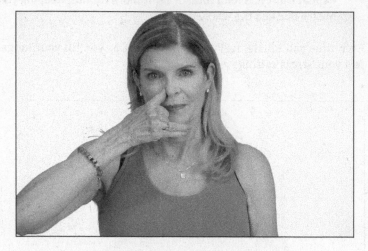

FIGURE 3-4: Alternate nostril breathing.

1. Sit comfortably on a chair or in one of the yogic sitting postures with your back straight.

2. Place your right hand so that your thumb is on the right nostril and the little and ring fingers are lightly on the left nostril, with the index and middle fingers tucked lightly into the hand (near the ball of the thumb).

3. Close the right nostril and inhale gently but fully through the left nostril — don't strain.

4. Open the right nostril and close the left, and exhale through the open nostril (right).

5. Inhale through the same nostril (right) then block that nostril and exhale through the left.

6. Repeat 10 to 15 times.

With practice, you can gradually increase the repetitions.

Bee breath

Bee breath is a particularly useful exercise for relieving anxiety, according to my friend and colleague Tim McCall. He wrote an entire article on this technique that appeared in the *Yoga Journal* (see "Bee Breath to Get Anxiety to Buzz Off," at www.yogajournal.com/practice/buzz-away-the-buzzing-mind). In the article, he explains that extending your exhale using this technique may trigger an immediate relaxation response. Additionally, you do make a bee-like sound in this routine, and the sound itself may be healing.

While doing the bee breath, don't force the sound or try too aggressively to extend your exhale, says McCall, or you may actually create even more anxiety.

1. Sit upright in a comfortable position.

2. Place your hands on your face with one thumb in each ear canal, your index and middle fingers on your eyes, your ring fingers closing your nostrils, and your pinky fingers on the corners of your mouth (see Figure 3-5).

   Use light pressure only, especially on your eyes.

3. Inhale completely through the nose.

4. As you exhale, make a humming sound in your throat.

5. Notice how you feel vibrations in your fingers.

6. Repeat for six to eight rounds.

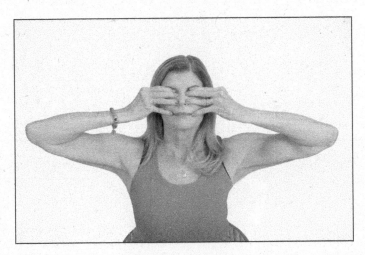

FIGURE 3-5:
Bee breath hand positions.

2

Yoga on the Mat

IN THIS PART . . .

Try a few Yoga postures.

Familiarize yourself with meditation, including various approaches.

Try a meditation exercise at home using step-by-step instructions.

Chapter 4

Twenty Great Postures for the 50-Plus Yogi

The obvious advantage of having a regular Yoga program is that it requires you to move in ways that you otherwise would not move during the course of a normal day. And by *movement*, I'm referring specifically to the stretching and strengthening that keeps your body flexible, straight, and strong, no matter your age.

But if Yoga is to be a benefit and help you become healthier, you have to practice in a way that keeps you free from injury. If you start practicing Yoga to become more fit and end up hurting yourself, you've already defeated the purpose.

Yoga needs to adapt to you and not the other way around. To that end, taking the time to learn the types of modifications you can choose as you bring your hard work to the mat will truly make all the difference.

Remembering Function over Form

I often use the expression "function over form," and that basically means that you should give top priority to how a particular Yoga pose serves you and your body and not be so worried about how it looks.

The postures I describe in this chapter are some of the most common in a Yoga practice — and they're also some of the safest, providing you modify them whenever needed.

REMEMBER

While you may receive numerous benefits from any given pose, including strengthening and stretching, your first objective is to enhance the health of your mind, as well as your spine.

But sometimes, for a pose to have the maximum positive impact, you need to choose a modification. It's always more important what a pose does for your body than what it looks like.

Listening to your body

Whether you're taking a class or practicing alone on your mat, keep in mind that you and you alone are in charge. Any good Yoga teacher will try to keep you safe. In fact, as I write this book, my first objective is to keep you safe. But, in the end, only you know what's going on inside your body at any given moment, so pay attention to how you're feeling.

This chapter highlights some of the most common poses in a Yoga practice. I present you with both the traditional form as well as the same pose with modifications. The modifications may actually make the pose more accessible and pain-free. Please don't see the modifications as doing less.

You should also take note that one side of your body may feel differently than the other. This is understandable, since no human is symmetrical and you're probably either right- or left-handed, which indicates your dominant side. Moreover, the things your body needs to stay healthy and safe may vary from one day to the next.

To modify or not to modify

I know that some movements or postures may be very easy for you, and you may choose to take a more traditional approach. Not everyone needs to modify every pose. Just don't be reluctant to modify any pose where needed. You may need to experiment a bit, just to see what feels best for your body. But please remember: "No pain, no gain" doesn't apply in Yoga. If something hurts, try a modification. If it still hurts, stop. Even some of the seemingly easiest poses still may not be good for your body structure. For example, even the simplest inversion may not benefit you if you have high blood pressure or retinopathy, are pregnant, or suffer from GERD.

As with any new physical activity, you should always consult your doctor before attempting any Yoga pose.

Focusing on the spine

You may have lost some ease of movement and grown a bit stiffer over time. One sign of this can be seen in your posture.

In the extreme, as muscles change, your spine may become less vertical, less straight (see Figure 4-1).

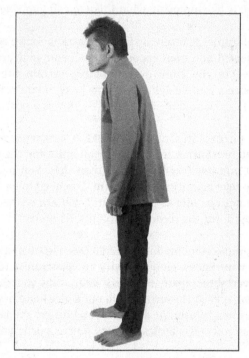

FIGURE 4-1: The spine becomes less erect.

That's why much of what I talk about in this book relates to the health of your spine. Even the Yoga poses I offer often have, as their primary objective, some love and care for your spine.

While you will certainly be strengthening some muscles in some poses and stretching and relaxing muscles in other poses, you will ultimately be standing straighter and walking taller as a result of adding Yoga to your routine.

For more information on your spine, see Chapters 10 and 11, including the sample home routines.

Forgiving limbs

The traditional form of a pose or traditional alignment should not be your most important consideration. If you try to force your body into a posture that you see in a book or on a nearby Yoga mat, you may be setting yourself up for injury.

REMEMBER

You need to be in a class, with a teacher, that allows you to let Yoga fit your body, to address exactly what you need at the moment. It makes no sense to force your body to fit a particular Yoga class.

The key, then, is to adapt Yoga to fit your body. I certainly help you with this adaptation as I look at specific poses. And one of the primary ways you are going to accomplish this goal is by employing what I like to call *forgiving limbs.*

Simply stated, the philosophy of forgiving limbs says that you're always, no matter what the pose, allowed and even encouraged to bend your arms and legs as needed. Bending prevents you from overstretching certain muscles (you can stretch a muscle or strain a muscle doing the same pose, if you're not thoughtful) and may allow you to keep your spine a bit erect — always a goal.

Yet, when you look at pictures in some Yoga books or magazine covers, everyone seems to have the straightest arms and legs — often imitating the very traditional form of the pose. But you need to be smarter than that. You need to allow the function of the pose to take priority over the form. You need to let Yoga serve you. In some cases, it may not be quite as pretty, but it will always be more effective, safer, even smarter. (And, for the record, I think just as pretty!)

Take, for example, a simple standing forward fold (see Figure 4-2). If you work to get your head toward your knees, giving gravity an opportunity to lengthen your spine and ease your vertebrae apart, it is very likely that your hamstrings (the back of your thighs) will object. However, if you put a nice bend in your knees, you will be able to get your head closer. As a result, you still get the benefit of letting the gravity decompress you — regardless of how much your knees are bent. This is *function over form.*

Fascia (or as I like to call it, your leotard)

Science describes *fascia* as a layer of connective tissue that runs throughout the body, supporting muscles, tendons, and organs. But I actually heard a colleague once refer to it as an internal "leotard." I like that description.

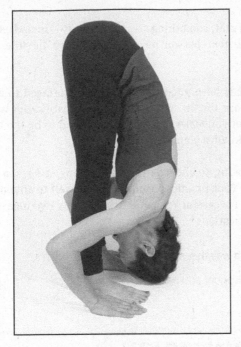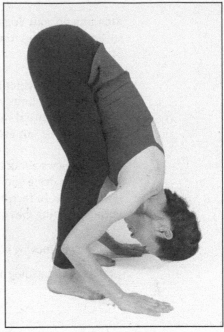

FIGURE 4-2:
Forward fold
(traditional and
modified).

Think of it as a one-piece suit that extends from somewhere in your feet, all the way up to somewhere in your head. It's important to be aware of this because things that happen in the bottom of your body can actually impact what's going on at the top.

As just one example, a pain you feel in your neck may be caused by something happening in, say, your ankle. Again, that's because of your leotard.

Keep in mind that your fascia likes to move and that it may be able to move more freely if you employ the forgiving limbs approach.

Yoga is not a competition

The first time some people began running around the school playground or participating in a spelling bee in the classroom, they experienced an innate desire to stand out, to be better than the next kid. The sense of competition seemed almost instinctive.

When it comes to Yoga, however, it's important to abandon any trace of a competitive nature.

Standing on your Yoga mat, something still inside you — inside us all —may want to be better than the next person on the mat. More flexible. More graceful. Stronger.

Perhaps this instinct has been good for you. Maybe the need to excel has served you well throughout your life, in school, in sports, at work. But when it comes to Yoga, it is essential that you learn to let go of that need to be the best. Yoga is not competitive — not even with yourself!

The good news about being 50 and over is that, perhaps, it's just a bit easier to not let your ego drive your Yoga practice. Comparing yourself to anyone else is a fruitless exercise. In fact, a successful Yoga practice has only two measures, illustrated in the following two questions:

>> Are you moving in a way that nurtures your body and spirit?

>> Are you avoiding all injury and pain?

MEN AND COMPETITION

Men in my classes seem particularly challenged by Yoga's noncompetitive nature. Over the years, they have often attempted to do the most challenging version of a pose, not because it's the right choice for their bodies, but because they want to compete with other men or impress the women in the class. Now, it may seem a bit inappropriate for me to make such a gender distinction, but it is nonetheless an accurate description of what I see in my classes.

This problem is even more obvious when the Yoga session is led by a (probably) hypermobile young woman. Too many men feel like they have to keep up with the instructor; and way too many men are injured in the attempt. (For more, see "Wounded Warrior Pose" in *The New York Times* at https://www.nytimes.com/2012/12/23/sunday-review/the-perils-of-yoga-for-men.html.)

One of the most common poses that leads to back injuries is the seated forward fold. I list that pose in Chapter 6, but pay particular attention to the suggested modifications. It would be great to send you to Appendix A for a complete list of all the prizes and certificates you can receive for getting into advanced poses. But there is no Appendix A; there are no prizes. Rather, your goals are to do what's smart for your body, stay safe, and forget about competing. Not getting hurt — now that's impressive!

Asymmetrical Forward Bend

The asymmetrical forward bend pose lengthens both the back and the hamstrings. This pose can be very challenging in its traditional form, particularly bringing your head toward your leg. You definitely don't want to ignore the most beneficial aspects of the pose by trying to make the pose look perfect.

TIP

Modification: Allow your forward leg to bend (instead of keeping it straight) to make it easier to stretch your back (see Figure 4-3). Notice in the modification how much closer the model can bring his torso to his leg just by bending his knee (see Figure 4-3), giving him more space to lengthen.

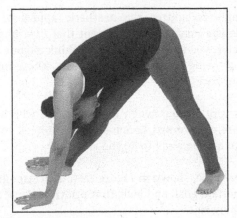 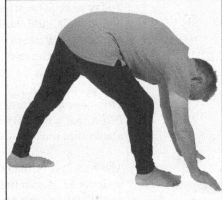

FIGURE 4-3:
Asymmetrical forward bend (traditional and modified).

Bent Leg Supine Twist

You will generally do twists toward the end of a Yoga sequence, when your muscles are warmed up and ready for stretching. The twisting posture continues strengthening and elongating those muscles that support your spine — all the way from the hips to the top of the spine.

This ultimately helps you stand straighter and walk more upright. Also, you prepare your back for sudden twisting movements that may happen when doing other things besides Yoga.

TIP

Modification: When you bring the bent knee across your body, the traditional form would require you to bring that knee to the floor (see Figure 4-4). Instead, bring that knee toward the floor only as far as you feel a stretch, but not pain.

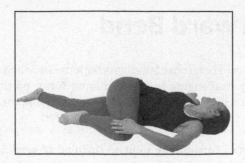
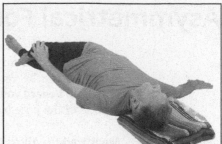

FIGURE 4-4:
Bent leg supine twist (traditional and modified).

Boat Pose

Today's society strongly recognizes the aesthetic appeal of well-developed abdominals. And while you may choose to accept that "washboard abs" are an established Western value, you should also start to think of your abdominal muscles, your entire core, as being the front of your spine. Those muscles do indeed provide support for your back.

This concept becomes very obvious when I treat people who have back issues. Often, back muscles are overworked because they're forced to do the work of abdominal muscles that are too weak to do the job.

The function of the boat pose, shown in Figure 4-5, is to strengthen the front of your spine. It's an important goal, and your first priority should not be how good you'll look in your bathing suit.

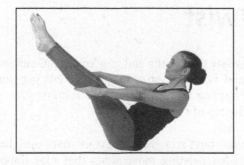
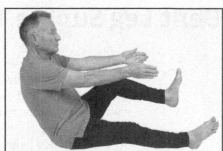

FIGURE 4-5:
Boat pose (traditional and modified).

TIP

Modification: While traditional boat pose is done with your legs straight (see Figure 4-5), one of the ways to modify it is to soften your knees. If this pose is still too challenging, trying lifting one leg while planting the other foot firmly on the mat (with your knee still bent). I include this pose here because it is a great way to build your core strength. It is critically important, however, for you to choose the appropriate modification (if needed).

Bridge Pose

Like so many postures, traditional Yoga equates numerous health benefits with the bridge pose. From insomnia and fatigue to anxiety and digestive issues, the bridge addresses a great deal.

For me, I primarily look at bridge pose variations as a way to compensate for abdominal work by integrating stability and control of the core.

In addition to compensating for abdominal work, bridge poses also prepare the neck and shoulder muscles for a shoulder stand inversion.

TIP

Modification: For some people, raising the hips off of the floor is too challenging. The easiest modification is to leave your hips on the ground, but tilt your pelvis upward (see Figure 4-6).

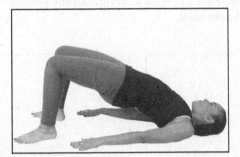 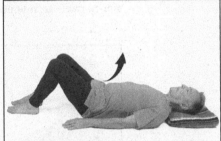

FIGURE 4-6:
Bridge pose (traditional and modified).

Child's Pose

For most people, child's pose is calming, and most Yoga classes will treat it as a resting pose (see Figure 4-7).

TIP

Modification: You can put your arms out in front of you or maybe alongside you (with your hands near your feet). Some people also find it easier to breathe if they open their knees instead of keeping them together.

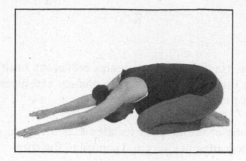
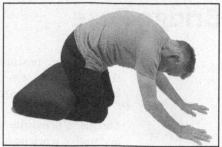

FIGURE 4-7:
Child's pose (traditional and modified).

Cobra Pose

Cobra pose is probably the most common back-bending posture (see Figure 4-8). The primary function of this pose is to lengthen and strengthen the spine. You also stretch your arms and shoulders as you push upward and let your shoulders fall back. In any form, you need to keep your hips on the ground — and be careful not to over-arch your lower back.

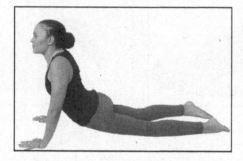
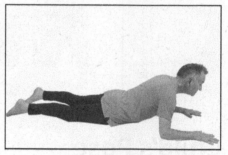

FIGURE 4-8:
Cobra pose (traditional and modified).

TIP

Modification: One of the first modifications I'd like to mention is keeping your gluteal muscles (your butt) loose. Your glutes are big muscles, and they will want to do all the work. If you keep them relaxed, you'll be forcing your low back muscles to take over instead. While the traditional cobra pose may allow you to use your gluteal muscles to help you lift, a more common technique requires you to keep your butt relaxed.

In Yoga therapy, we help restore the natural lumbar curve in the lower back using the cobra pose without activating the gluteals. With too much sitting becoming the new smoking, adversely impacting general health, we use this technique more and more.

Also note in the modified version shown in Figure 4-7 the model is doing this pose on his forearms (often called sphinx arms). This modification may be a good place to start if this pose is new to you.

Corpse Pose

Corpse pose (see Figure 4-9) is a relaxation pose that is always a real favorite — especially at the end of a class or home session. Yet it's still a Yoga pose, so you need to remember that at least some work needs to be done.

The primary function of corpse pose is rest. This pose is sometimes used at the beginning of class to help you relax and turn your attention away from what happened earlier or what may be on your agenda for later — or maybe just the grocery list. It's a pose that gives you an opportunity to steady your mind and connect with your breath.

FIGURE 4-9: Corpse pose (traditional and modified).

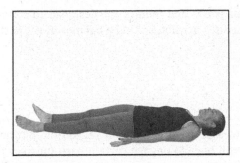 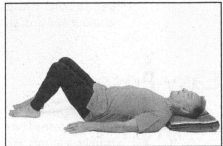

At the end, the pose gives you an opportunity to make sure that you have relaxed all the muscles you used throughout the practice and once again find a place inside that is peaceful and stress-free.

Modification: The primary goal of this pose is to be comfortable, so feel free to make any adjustments that will help you relax. A common modification is to bend the knees with support.

TIP

Downward Facing Dog

Like so many postures, the downward facing dog (Figure 4-10) Yoga pose (see Figure 4-10) offers a multitude of benefits. Still, the lengthening of the spine as it slightly arches as well as the hamstrings is readily apparent.

Modification: The problem with this pose is that you can put too much weight in your hands, creating issues for your wrists and shoulders. Bending your knees can help you distribute your weight more evenly and maybe even allow you to lower your heels closer to the ground. You could also try walking your feet slightly closer to your hands.

TIP

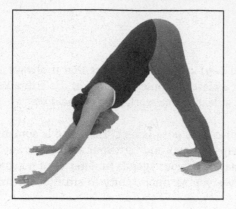
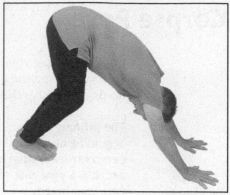

FIGURE 4-10:
Downward facing dog pose (traditional and modified).

Keep in mind that your pelvis and femurs are designed to support your weight. Shoulder and arm structures are not, so find a balance of support.

Easy Pose

WARNING

The easy pose Figure (4-11) is clearly used for relaxation. But beware that, to sit straight and tall, you will have to engage certain back muscles that will actually strengthen as you hold the pose.

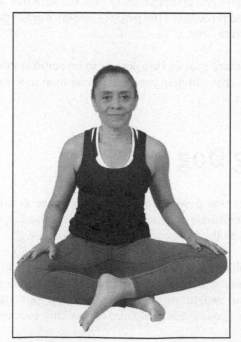
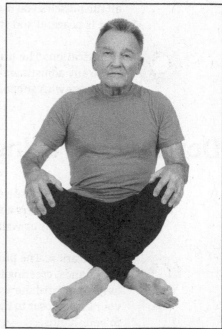

FIGURE 4-11:
Easy pose (traditional and modified).

One school of thought in Yoga philosophy believes all Yoga postures are designed to stabilize your body so that you will be stable enough to sit in this position for long periods of time — particularly for meditation.

Modification: If you want to make this pose easier, especially if you're staying in it for a few minutes, it helps to sit on something. It could be a stack of blankets, blocks, a bolster, or a cushion. Elevating your spine helps make it longer without using your own muscles to do it. You can also sit against a wall to support your back.

TIP

Great Seal

In traditional Yoga, the great seal pose (see Figure 4-12) is generally considered advanced because it requires doing all three of the locks or *bandhas*, as they're called in traditional Yoga. In Sanskrit, *bandha* means to tighten or hold tight. I am including this pose in this chapter because its modified version offers a great way to relax and to strengthen the back muscles and the rest of the core.

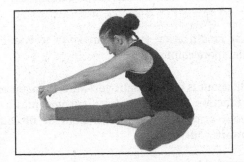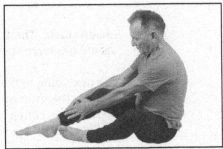

FIGURE 4-12:
Great seal pose
(traditional and
modified).

Modification: In this more accessible version of the pose, don't add the locks (at least not right away). It still yields great benefits. Notice that in the modified version, you can soften the knee of the straight leg.

TIP

Half Chair Pose

In a traditional chair or half chair pose (see Figure 4-13), your arms and legs are stretching and strengthening, which happens in the modified version as well (though, maybe to a lesser extent). But it's the extension of the spine that is the primary function.

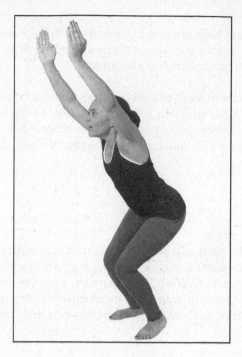
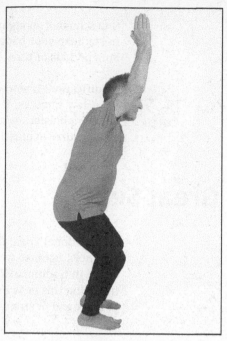

TIP

Modification: The first modification you can make is to widen your stance. It should feel more stable, more comfortable.

The next thing to think about is how straight you want to make your arms. Again, because the primary function of this pose is to put you into a slight backbend (extension), soften your arms if you feel any pain or discomfort when you straighten them up toward your ears.

Finally, pay attention to how your knees feel and decide how deeply you want to squat. Because it is a half chair pose, even the traditional version will go down only halfway. You may decide that, for you at that moment, less than halfway makes more sense.

Half-Standing Forward Bend

Once again, the function of the half-standing forward bend pose (see Figure 4-14) relates to the spine. In each version of the pose, the back is slightly arched. Holding this pose not only lengthens and strengthens the back muscles, but it also targets the arms and shoulders.

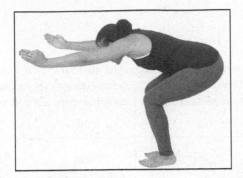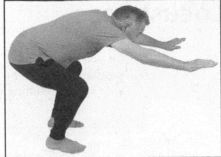

FIGURE 4-14:
Half-standing
forward bend
pose (traditional
and modified).

TIP

Modification: Putting a slight bend in the arms makes this pose more accessible while still allowing for a slightly arched back. Also, notice that the feet are wider in the modified pose (instead of together), making for a more comfortable, sturdier stance.

Knees-to-Chest

While the knees-to-chest resting pose may seem very basic, it is an important way to compensate the body after doing back bends and twists. It is a reset, of sorts, and a great way to massage your lower back (especially if you rock side to side). Bending your knees takes pressure off the back of your legs and lumbar area (see Figure 4-15).

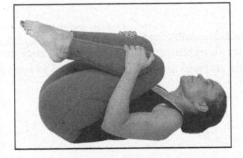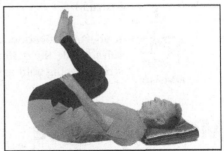

FIGURE 4-15:
Knees-to-chest
pose (traditional
and modified).

TIP

Modification: One of the ways you can modify this pose is by positioning your hands behind your knees instead of in front of them or putting them on your knee caps with arms extended.

Locust Pose

All you need to do is look at the photographs to know that the locust pose is primarily a back bend (see Figure 4-16). You have to use the muscles supporting your spine, including your gluteal muscles, to achieve an arch in your back.

FIGURE 4-16:
Locust pose
(traditional and
modified).

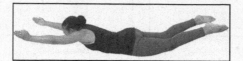
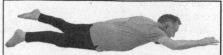

TIP

Modifications: You have the choice of several variations or modifications in this pose. Most of them have to do with what you do with your arms and legs. Modifications include

>> Both legs on the ground

>> One leg on the ground and lifting the other

>> Both arms in front of you, remaining on the ground as you lift

>> One arm lifts while the other remains down

>> One or both arms down at your sides

You should try various combinations in this pose to see what works best for you at the moment. (Don't strain your back by trying to create a bigger arch: Think long instead.)

REMEMBER

If your modification includes using just one arm and/or leg, be sure to do both sides. While the primary function of the pose may be a back bend, you're also strengthening your arms and legs as you lift, so you need to keep both sides even.

Mountain Pose

Mountain pose is often used as a starting position. As you can see, it is a relatively easy pose, but keep in mind it should also be a strong pose — your muscles are engaged, even strengthened in the process (see Figure 4-17).

If, however, your first priority in any posture is thinking about what it's doing for your spine, this pose is no different. To that end, mountain pose is an opportunity for you to stand straight and tall, to improve and maybe even train your posture.

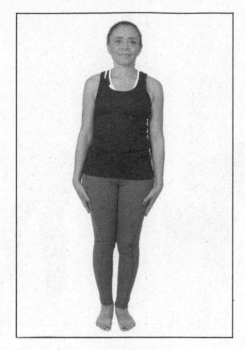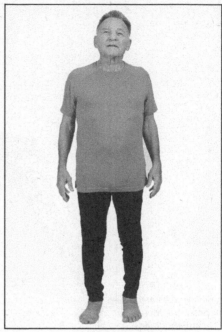

FIGURE 4-17: Mountain pose (traditional and modified).

TIP

Modification: One modification you can make in this pose is to bring your feet to about hips-width apart, instead of standing in the more traditional way with your feet together. Bringing your palms forward requires your shoulders to open and to stretch your upper chest muscles (pectorals). Palms at your side is more relaxed.

Try this posture with and without modifications to decide what feels best.

Revolved Triangle

Twisting poses like the revolved triangle have many reputed benefits in Yoga, but the primary function in this pose is the lengthening of the back muscles (see Figure 4-18). Like all twists, this pose can provide some relief for low back pain — depending, of course, on what's causing the pain.

TIP

Modification: The first way to modify this pose (as shown in the Figure 4-18) is to put as much bend in your knees as feels comfortable. Just doing that will help you go into your twist. Additionally, if you can't reach the floor. . .

Also, if it's painful for you to reach upward, you can also wrap your hand around your low back (still keeping your shoulder up toward the ceiling).

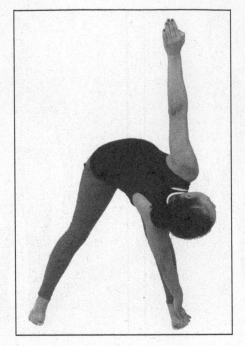
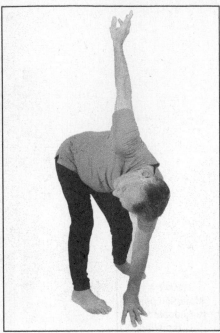

FIGURE 4-18:
Revolved triangle pose (traditional and modified).

Seated Forward Bend

The seated forward bend pose (see Figure 4-19) is great for lengthening the spine and surrounding shoulder muscles, and traditional Yoga even notes benefits relating to digestion, weight loss, anxiety, and insomnia. But another important, less positive result of this pose is injury.

The goal is to bring your head toward your knees. But, most people's hamstrings will prevent that from happening.

WARNING

All too often, people try to compensate for tight hamstrings by increasing the bend using their spines, which may lead to a back injury. You need to be thoughtful when doing this pose.

TIP

Modification: The first modification you can make is to bend your knees. Again, the function of the pose doesn't relate to the legs — not even the hamstrings (even though they'll be challenged). If the focus is on the spine, bending your knees will allow you to bend forward more. If it feels okay, you can round your back; if it hurts to round, keep your back long.

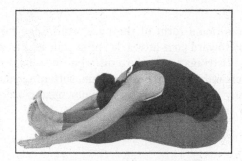

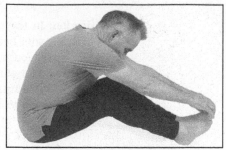

FIGURE 4-19: Seated forward bend (traditional and modified).

Standing Forward Bend

All day long, as you sit or stand, walk or drive, you remain upright, with gravity pulling your vertebrae together — in effect, compressing your spine (your discs are designed to help cushion that compression). The goal of the standing forward bend pose (see Figure 4-20) is actually to decompress your spine. You can see that the pull of gravity spreads your vertebrae apart. Your spine is lengthened and decompressed.

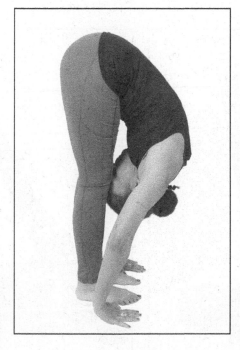

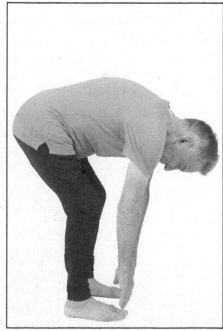

FIGURE 4-20: Standing forward bend pose (traditional and modified).

Modification: In the traditional form of the pose, you hinge forward from the hips, bringing your head toward your knees, keeping your legs as straight as possible. Of course, your hamstrings may have a different idea. Because the function of the pose is to lengthen and decompress the spine, softening your knees (bending your legs) is a totally acceptable way to get your head closer to your knees. Don't worry about your tight hamstrings.

TIP

Supported Shoulder Stand

Doing inverted poses in Yoga addresses many purported problems, including insomnia, digestion problems, menopause symptoms, and anxiety. From my experience, the issue is that inversions are the category of Yoga poses that causes the most injuries. The challenge is to find a version of the pose that is relatively safe, while still offering the benefits.

The primary reason I include the supported shoulder stand (see Figure 4-21) is that it offers most of the benefits of an inversion, while at the same time is safer than the more advanced inversions.

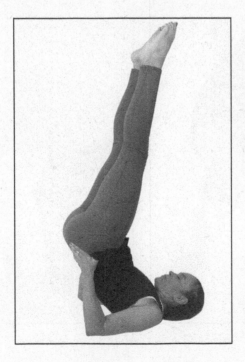 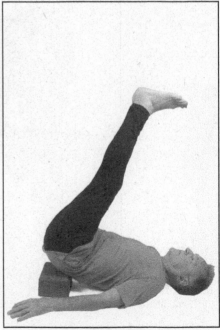

FIGURE 4-21: Supported shoulder stand (traditional and modified).

TIP

Modification: Deleting this since we're saying it above. You can use any number of props, including a bolster, foam block, or stack of blankets, under your lower back to lift your hips. (If the pose is still too challenging, try putting your legs up a wall.)

In a Yoga class, you often hear about reversing blood flow, but you know that your blood always flows in the same direction. You are, however, reversing the impact of gravity on your circulation. When you're inverted, gravity helps direct the blood back to your heart, making your heart work less to get it there and ultimately helping you to relax more.

Warrior I

Like so many Yoga poses, the Warrior I pose (see Figure 4-22) has numerous benefits. You're strengthening the front of the thigh (quadricep) of your forward leg and stretching the back of your other leg. But, as always, it's what's happening in your spine that is the most important aspect of this pose.

Coming into this pose requires you to arch your back. The muscles in your back that are supporting your spine are activated and strengthened.

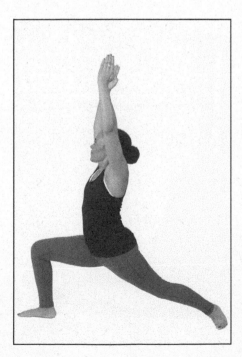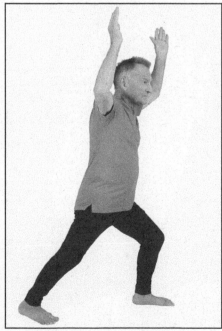

FIGURE 4-22:
Warrior I pose
(traditional and
modified).

TIP

Modification: How much you choose to straighten or bend your limbs is entirely up to you. If you need to bend your arms more or perhaps bend your legs less, make that choice — particularly if such modifications help you arch your back. Of course, if activating any of these muscles causes you pain, then bending a bit forward will allow you to find some relief and hopefully maintain some version of the pose.

Chapter **5**

Meditation for the 50-Plus Mind

My primary teacher from India, T.K.V. Desikachar, offered a lecture on meditation in San Diego around 2001. When asked to define the difference between prayer and meditation, he said, "Prayer is when you talk to God; meditation is when you listen." Even if you don't believe in God or are in no way religious, meditation is a great thing!

Benefiting from Meditation

Certainly, meditation has its roots in various religious and spiritual traditions, but it has evolved into something more.

Even the term meditation is hard to define, mostly because it means so many things to so many different people, cultures, religions, and even Yoga lineages. Yet it's imperative to talk about meditation in this book because when it comes to Yoga, exercising your mind is every bit as important as exercising your body. And, of course, Yoga does both. Meditation in that sense is not mystical, but rather very practical.

The health benefits of meditation are numerous and signficant:

» Reduced blood pressure

» Less anxiety and stress

» Better circulation

» Deeper relaxation

» Better sleep

» Better control of pain management

» Lower heart rate

» Slower respiratory rate

» Decrease in cortisol levels (stress hormone)

» Increase in endorphins (feel-good hormone)

There's also what I call a spiritual benefit for those people who practice meditation as part of a religious tradition or even Yoga.

In fact, if you look at some of the early Yogic texts, meditation is presented as a tool to achieve enlightenment or to find spiritual bliss. While I don't want to discount this aspect of meditation, I focus instead on ways to achieve the health benefits. I leave you to discover any deeper benefits during your own personal journey.

Steady the Mind

So many news and magazine articles and studies by major universities have highlighted the clinical evidence that supports all the health benefits related to meditation that I probably don't even need to sell you on the practice. But if you still need convincing, it seems like every major medical and scientific source you can turn to will support my contention.

A study "Mindfulness practice leads to increases in regional brain gray matter density," Volume 191, Issue 1, 30 January 2011, Pages 36–43 published in *Psychiatry Research: Neuroimaging* found that older adults who meditated experienced changes in their gray matter and ultimately had brains that structurally resembled young adults. (Those older adults who didn't meditate did not experience the same neurological tranformation.) The implications are profound.

And, as complex as these results may seem, the actual process of meditation is much more straightforward. While you should celebrate the fact that your mind is capable of *multitasking* — thinking of many things at once — the goal of meditation is to turn it down. Way down.

As I'm lying on my Yoga mat or sitting upright in a chair, I may be having angry thoughts about the guy who cut me off on the highway this morning. At the same time, I might also be worrying about a meeting with my boss or partner later on today.

My mind is partially in the past — and I'm probably producing stress hormones as I mentally confront that inconsiderate driver from this morning. But I'm also in the future, thinking about that stressful meeting I have coming up, and my shoulders are getting tight in anticipation. My mind is everywhere at once, except in the present moment.

But the present moment is your goal. Let your attention be in the here and now. Probably most of your stress comes from thinking about what's already happened or what may happen. Your brain is ready to respond with chemicals like adreneline or cortisol — hormones that will help you stay and fight or just run from trouble. The way to keep these chemicals out of your bloodstream is to keep your mind in the present moment. Of course, that's easier said than done.

Yet each one of the meditation techniques I cover in this chapter attempts to do just that. The idea is to learn to focus your mind on something — probably on one thing. Once you learn to keep your attention steady, everything changes in your body.

Types of Meditation

If you decide to explore meditation, your next task is to decide what technique works for you — and not everything will. It's not only okay to try something and then set it aside because it's not working for you, but that's actually part of the process.

Like Yoga, meditation must fit the individual, and you may need to explore several approaches before finding one that's right for you. The following sections describe several meditation styles or traditions.

Yoga postures

Think of Yoga postures as a moving meditation. Your body benefits from the stretching and strengthening, while you give your mind something to focus on as you pay attention to every breath, in every posture.

Meditation has been clinically proven to help manage pain or stress. So many things are happening in your body at any given moment: Your heart is beating, your blood is flowing through your veins, you're probably digesting your last meal. But all those things are hard to feel. Yet breathing — the inhaling and exhaling — is quite easy to feel, quite easy to direct your mental focus on. (See Chapter 3 for more about breathing.)

Mindfulness meditation

The term *mindfulness* is pervasive today and on the top of the list when it comes to popular approaches to meditation. Mindfulness has a rich history, with its roots in Buddhism, and then a profound emergence in academic and scientific circles, and finally into the mainstream of Western life. Meditation can bring your thoughts out of the past and the future and into the present (or as the Yoga cliché calls it, into the moment). Mindfulness really has the same goal, asking you to bring your attention — perhaps using all of your senses — to what's happening around you right now. Doing this technique is a way of being mindful, and you can potentially practice it anywhere, from sitting on a cushion or a Yoga mat to drinking a cup of tea or standing in line at the supermarket.

Transcendental meditation

Sometimes referred to as TM, *transcendental meditation* is an approach that gained popularity during the 1960s with people like The Beatles. The TM movement has gained a lot of popularity over the decades, though the organization itself is highly regulated and the technique is taught by certified teachers within the organization itself, usually for a fee.

TM uses a *mantra* (a phrase mentally recited over and over again), giving your mind something on which to focus. While my own experience with TM is somewhat limited, I found it to be powerful. Moreover, the anecdotal response over the years has also been quite favorable.

REMEMBER

Keep in mind that the use of a mantra in meditation works great for some people, but not so great for others.

Loving-kindness meditation (metta meditation)

In a study of middle-aged adults with no meditation experience, loving-kindness meditation showed significant results. I think the title of an article published in the journal *Psychoneuroendocrinology* (October 2019) says it all: "Loving-kindness meditation slows biological aging in novices: Evidence from a 12-week randomized controlled trial."

The study involved 176 subjects who were assigned a meditation practice (either a mindful meditation routine or a loving-kindness routine), or they remained on a wait list and did not meditate at all. The team of doctors and scientists that conducted the study talked about the difference between people's chronological age and their biological age. Your chronological age is simply expressed by how long you've been on the planet. It's measured in years. Your biological age, however, is frequently measured, at least by scientists, in "telomere length."

I don't want to get too technical, but telomeres are found on each of your DNA chromosomes and they tend to shorten over time. What the study found was that the telomeres of people practicing a loving-kindness meditation did not shorten. This simple form of meditation may actually change you on the cellular level.

The relationship between the brain and meditation remains a topic of a lot of research, but the other development observed by the team that conducted the study is that those people practicing the loving-kindness meditation developed more compassion and affection toward the people in their lives.

The study's implications are obviously significant. While mindfulness tries to focus the mind in a nonjudgmental way on what's happening in the present, the loving-kindness technique leads you toward developing feelings of love and compassion for yourself and the people around you.

Later in this chapter, I include an example of the loving-kindness meditation.

Guided meditation

As you may guess, *guided meditation* typically involves being led by a teacher or facilitator who may be in the same room or on an app, recording device, or website. In any case, your focus is on the voice of the person leading the meditation.

I include guided meditation here because, to me, it offers two very important features:

>> **It gives your mind a place to focus.** Instead of tuning your senses to the world around you or mentally reciting a mantra, you simply focus your attention on the speaker — on your *guide*.

>> **This type of meditation focuses on the words themselves.** If you thoughtfully select the topic of your meditation, you may hear words or thoughts that you really need to hear. Maybe the guide is going to help you affirm things about yourself or the world around you, or maybe the guide is going to take you somewhere: in nature, back in time, or inside your body.

Guided meditations can be powerful, and you may want to try a few to see if you like them. Many are available for free.

Kirtan Kriya

Kirtan Kriya is not as well-known as the other types of meditation, but it's becoming more and more prominent — particularly because of studies looking into how it may strengthen or heal cognitive performance. And if you think you may not be as mentally sharp as you were when you were younger, this technique is worth exploring.

The Alzheimer's Research and Prevention Foundation is researching this specific type of meditation, noting improvements in brain function for those who practice it. Indeed, I've read about this type of meditation in *Psychology Today* and the *Yoga Journal*, so it seemed important to include it here.

The practice of Yoga is often broken down by lineage. This type of meditation is from the Kundalini tradition. It uses both mantra and mudras (hand positions). Later in this chapter, I include a step-by-step process for you to try.

Meditation Routines for Home

As you've seen, meditation has many health benefits, so I'd certainly recommend the practice to anyone of any age. The goal, of course, is to find a meditation approach that works for you.

I highlight three techniques not only because they're relatively easy to do, but because some impressive research suggests that these techniques offer positive cognitive effects for 50-plus practitioners.

Mindful meditation routine

Turn to Chapter 8, where I share with you a body scan technique that can be described as a form of mindful meditation because it asks you to assess your body in the present moment.

In that routine, I give you written instructions for performing a body scan on yourself, asking you how various parts of your body feel at the moment. As you do this body scan, I want you to keep two things in mind:

>> The instructions can easily be presented to you as part of a guided meditation, led by someone physically in the room, as well as by someone who was previously recorded.

>> While all forms of meditation may give your mind something to focus on (or perhaps ask you not to focus on anything), the mind is not necessarily going to cooperate. For your entire life, your mind has served you well by thinking of many things at once. Don't expect that pattern of thinking to be easily changed.

TIP

My advice to you is accept your intruding thoughts — even treasure them. Then, let them go. Meditation takes practice, and even using techniques like those I describe here, the mind will still jump around. Don't shoot for perfection, just shoot for moments of focus. Even fleeting moments mark progress.

Loving-kindness meditation

You can practice the loving-kindness meditation in several ways, but I recommend that you first focus on yourself:

1. **Find a comfortable, seated position.**

   You can sit cross-legged on your Yoga mat or upright in a chair. The key word, here, is comfort. You could even be lying down, but why risk falling asleep?

REMEMBER

2. **Close your eyes and begin focused breathing, inhaling and exhaling (through the nose, only, if possible).**

3. **Imagine that with each inhale, you're taking in a healing or nurturing breath; with every exhale, imagine negative energy or illness leaving your body.**

4. **Mentally, say to yourself:**

   - May I be happy.

   - May I be healthy.

   - May I be safe.

   - May I be peaceful and at ease.

5. **Repeat these words to yourself, at least three more times (or as many times as you want if you like the feeling).**

6. **Silently, notice how these words make you feel; dwell in a moment of love and compassion.**

7. **At the end of your meditation, remember the way it made you feel.**

   You can carry that feeling with you throughout the day and use it when needed.

Note: While some may argue that you must first show love and kindness to yourself before you're truly able to wish it for others, feel free to continue this meditation by turning your compassion toward others. Your family may first come to mind, but also think of the broader world — or even someone you don't really like:

>> May <u>you</u> be happy.

>> May <u>you</u> be healthy.

>> May <u>you</u> be safe.

>> May <u>you</u> be peaceful and at ease.

You can go through this mediation as many times as you like, with as many different people. You may want to conclude the meditation by including everyone at once, even yourself:

>> May <u>we</u> be happy.

>> May <u>we</u> be healthy.

>> May <u>we</u> be safe.

>> May <u>we</u> be peaceful and at ease.

Kirtan Kriya routine

In this chapter, I share the techniques that have some clinical studies behind them and that have proven to be particularly effective for people who are 55 and older. The Kirtan Kriya meditation falls into that category, and you can do it in just 12 minutes.

This meditation uses sound and the vibration of that sound in the body. The placement of the tongue on the roof of the mouth to make certain sounds is a critical part of the meditation. It actually uses four easy words:

>> Saa (birth)

>> Taa (life)

>> Naa (death)

>> Maa (rebirth)

Also, musical notes are associated with each word, but, again, it's easy. Just think of each word as having the same note as *Mary Had a Little Lamb*:

> Mar—y—had—a
>
> Saa—Taa—Naa—Maa

That's the tune — just four notes!

Finally, there are hand mudras, which basically refers to certain ways to position the hand or move the fingers that, traditionally speaking, alter or adjust the way energy flows through the body. Like sound, these mudras are an essential part of the meditation technique (see Figure 5-1).

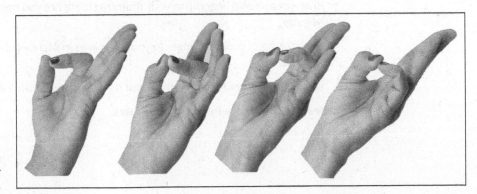

FIGURE 5-1:
Hand mudras for
Kirtan Kriya.

To begin:

1. **Sit in a comfortable cross-legged position on the floor, your Yoga mat, or on a cushion (or sit tall in a chair).**

2. **Rest your hands on your knees, palms up.**

3. **Using both hands (as they gently rest on your knees or thighs), complete the following sequence:**

   - Bring your index fingertip to your thumb as you sing *Saa*.

   - Bring your middle fingertip to your thumb as you sing *Taa*.

   - Bring the tip of your ring finger to your thumb as you sing *Naa*.

   - Bring the tip of your little finger to your thumb as you sing *Maa*.

4. **Repeat this sequence for about 2 minutes.**

5. **Using both hands (as they gently rest on your knees or thighs), complete the following sequence:**

   - Bring your index fingertip to your thumb as you whisper *Saa*.

   - Bring your middle fingertip to your thumb as you whisper *Taa*.

   - Bring the tip of your ring finger to your thumb as you whisper *Naa*.

   - Bring the tip of your little finger to your thumb as you whisper *Maa*.

6. **Repeat this sequence for about 2 minutes.**

7. **Using both hands (as they gently rest on your knees or thighs), complete the following sequence:**

   - Bring your index fingertip to your thumb as in silence you mentally sing *Saa*.

   - Bring your middle fingertip to your thumb as in silence you mentally sing *Taa*.

   - Bring the tip of your ring finger to your thumb as in silence you mentally sing *Naa*.

   - Bring the tip of your little finger to your thumb as you whisper *Maa*.

8. **Repeat this sequence for about 4 minutes.**

9. Using both hands (as they gently rest on your knees or thighs), complete the following sequence:

- Bring your index fingertip to your thumb as you whisper *Saa.*

- Bring your middle fingertip to your thumb as you whisper *Taa.*

- Bring the tip of your ring finger to your thumb as you whisper *Naa.*

- Bring the tip of your little finger to your thumb as you whisper *Maa.*

10. Repeat this sequence for about 2 minutes.

11. Using both hands (as they gently rest on your knees or thighs), complete the following sequence:

- Bring your index fingertip to your thumb as you sing *Saa.*

- Bring your middle fingertip to your thumb as you sing *Taa.*

- Bring the tip of your ring finger to your thumb as you sing *Naa.*

- Bring the tip of your little finger to your thumb as you sing *Maa.*

12. Repeat this sequence for about 2 minutes.

3

Yoga in Your Everyday Life

IN THIS PART . . .

Find easy ways to integrate healthy eating into your life.

Recognize the power behind the way you think.

Learn how Yoga can help you get a better night's sleep.

Chapter **6**

Yoga, Your Food, and Your Weight

Many people struggle with their weight. If you fall into that category, or if you're interested in maintaining a healthy diet, this chapter is for you.

While Yoga philosophy offers limited guidance on diet and nutrition, as a Yoga therapist, I've been counseling students, clients, and patients for many years. I've also traveled the world and spoken to great Yoga masters. So I definitely have some advice to share.

But I'm not a trained nutritionist or dietician, and I highly recommend you work with one. Specialists are in a much better position to give you personal guidance. And what could be more important than what you eat? Even if you're not dealing with excess weight, your food still represents your nourishment and ultimately helps determine your overall health.

Reaping the Benefits of a Balanced Diet

There's probably nothing you do in your day-to-day life that is more driven by habit than eating. Since the minute you came into this world, you wanted food, and many of us develop eating patterns that have been with us for a lifetime.

The problem is the way of eating you developed as a child may not always serve you well today.

Yoga philosophy doesn't offer a lot of guidance on the best foods to eat, and even Yoga therapists should not provide you with an approach that would be better coming from trained nutritionists and other medical professionals. That said, Yoga does recognize that as you age, you require a few hundred less calories a day, or you may notice your weight creeping up.

REMEMBER

Most people can't continue to eat in the same way they did as teenagers.

So, it does make sense to acknowledge what even Yoga masters have said: "Eat less as you get older." As I briefly provide you with a Yoga perspective on eating and weight management, keep two essential things in mind:

>> Yoga teachers and Yoga therapists are not nutritionists. Consider talking with a trained professional when trying to identify the best food plan for you.

>> There is a difference between weight loss and nutrition. If you're trying to address one, your goal should be to not compromise the other.

You do not need to be a vegetarian

The issue of Yoga and vegetarianism is one that has been debated for a long time. I am well aware that some interpretations of Yoga philosophy require dedicated Yoga practitioners to be vegetarians. I am equally aware, however, that nutritional needs are very unique.

While people can always debate the interpretation of the ancient Yoga texts that address this topic, I am reluctant to make judgments about who is and who isn't a dedicated practitioner of Yoga, based on their diets. Instead, you should discover the benefits of a Yoga practice while walking your own path.

REMEMBER

Only you (and perhaps your nutritionist) should decide what are the best foods for you. You may find it helpful to read *Ayurveda For Dummies* (Wiley) by Angela Hope-Murray.

One food plan does not fit all

In today's world, people are inundated with advertisements for the perfect diet. Everyone claims to have the perfect weight management solution. The problem is that the perfect diet for you isn't necessarily the perfect diet for me.

I tell you throughout this book that your Yoga practice has to be right for you. Why? Because you are unique, your body is unique, and your nutritional needs are unique. One-size-fits-all Yoga is not a smart approach — and neither is a one-size-fits-all diet.

Some diets work for some people, and some don't. That's why the best thing you can do is find out what you need. Do you have any vitamin deficiencies, food allergies, or food sensitivities? This information is important to have — and, again, not information you would get from your Yoga teacher.

I am confident, however, that if you have issues with weight gain (as many do), eating a little less will not jeopardize your health, so I will stand by that advice.

Stress eating

Not only have I personally experienced stress-related eating throughout the years, but talking with other diet experts confirmed it: Stress and anxiety often lead to overeating or compulsive eating. You probably already know that.

It may seem odd to you that people who start meditating or practicing Yoga (which can be considered a moving meditation) often start to lose weight. The explanation is simple: Yoga causes the body to relax and, as a result, reduce its production of *cortisol,* a stress-related hormone. Cortisol is associated with weight gain, and the reduction of cortisol can help with weight loss.

Yoga is a reliable tool for controlling stress and can, as a result, reduce compulsive or emotional eating.

Smartphone apps

A number of smartphone apps make following an eating plan even easier. I mention a few that have worked for some of my students, and they may help you as well:

>> **Fooducate** (www.fooducate.com): Track what you eat and see how healthy your food is.

>> **Lose it** (www.loseit.com): Track your food intake and activities to help you reach weight goals.

>> **MyFitnessPal** (www.myfitnesspal.com): Track your diet and exercise to calculate calorie goals.

You can research these and other apps to decide whether any of them might be a useful tool for you. You can use them to track both your calories (a big one for me) and your nutritional intake.

Don't Forget the Cardio

REMEMBER

The style of Yoga I focus on in this book isn't a form of cardio exercise. Yet most trainers will tell you that you need to add some cardio to your routine — not only to burn some extra calories, but also to keep your heart healthy.

While many of the flow classes or power Yoga classes are so fast moving that they get your heart rate up, those classes aren't for everyone. If you need other ways to supplement your Yoga routine to get your cardio workout, try these at a pace that raises your heartrate:

>> Walking outdoors or on a treadmill

>> Using the elliptical machine

>> Biking outdoors or on a stationary bike, at home or in a class

>> Swimming

There are, of course, other options, but these are no- or low-impact.

At its inception, Yoga was not intended to be a cardio workout, although there are many exceptions today. But the Yoga described in this book is designed to do in a relaxed state, with your heart beating at a resting rate.

Practicing Yoga while Seated

While you may be very capable of benefiting from the Yoga routines I provide in this book, I designed this 15-minute seated sequence for those hindered by excessive weight or those stuck behind a desk all day. I call it Desk Yoga or Executive Yoga. This specific routine is designed to get you moving without doing any excessive folding (which may be uncomfortable for some people).

Sometimes, when you see Yoga being done from a chair, the practice itself may seem watered down. This couldn't be further from the truth. Any type of movement can be a powerful tool, and you move plenty in this sequence.

WARNING

Nothing in this routine should cause you pain. If something does or even if your intuition tells you it's not a good idea to comply, then please don't. Again, nobody knows better how you're feeling than you.

Prepare for either of these routines by sitting in a chair with your back straight and your hands on your thighs. If it feels okay, close your eyes (or maybe just look at the floor).

Begin to shift your focus from events that have already happened or from items on your schedule for later to a quiet place inside. Try to link your body, breath, and mind. Again, that's what makes this Yoga and not just another exercise routine.

Breathe through your nose, inhaling and exhaling, with your mouth closed (if possible). Every time you exhale, gently draw your belly in. I call this *focus breathing*.

Now, picture your alignment, with your ear, shoulder, and hip in one straight line (see Figure 6-1).

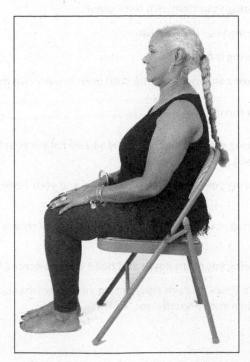

FIGURE 6-1:
Proper alignment.

Form a clear intention to relax and try to maintain this focus breathing throughout the sequence.

Fifteen-minute routine

I designed this routine specifically for my clients who found traditional Yoga routines to be inconsistent with their particular body type (and I'm talking about both men and women) as well as those sitting in an office too many hours a day. My hope is that you'll find the time to do the full routine (it should take you only about 15 minutes). Again, it's structured for you to do most of the work while in your chair. After you go down to the mat, you need to do only a couple of poses on your back before you move into some constructive rest.

If, however, you're constrained by time, I recommend the truncated version of the routine in the following section. It should take only about 5 minutes, and something is always better than nothing.

Arm raises:

TIP

1. **As you inhale, bring your right arm overhead (see Figure 6-2).**

   A soft bend in the elbow may make it more comfortable.

2. **As you exhale, bring your right arm back down.**

3. **As you inhale, bring your left arm up.**

4. **As you exhale, bring it down.**

5. **Continue the same sequence, moving with your breath two more times.**

Arm raises with head turn:

1. **As you inhale, bring your right arm overhead and rotate your head to the left (see Figure 6-3).**

2. **As you exhale, bring your right arm back down and your head back to center.**

3. **As you inhale, bring your left arm up and let your head rotate to the right.**

4. **As you exhale, bring your arm down and head back to center.**

5. **Repeat two more times on each side, timing your movement with your natural inhalations and exhalations.**

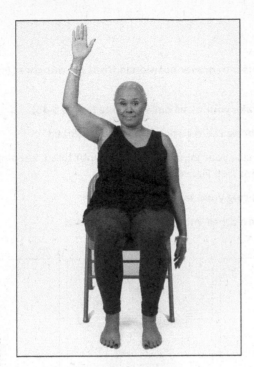

FIGURE 6-2:
Arm raises.

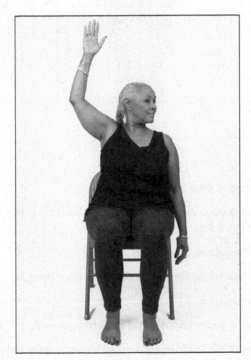

FIGURE 6-3:
Arm raises with
head turns.

Wing and prayer:

1. **Bring your hands into prayer position in front of your chest (see Figure 6-4a).**

2. **As you inhale, take your arms out wide (see Figure 6-4b).**

3. **As you exhale, bring them back to where you started.**

4. **As you inhale, raise your joined hands over your head, keeping your eyes on your fingertips (see Figure 6-4c).**

5. **As you exhale, bring your arms back down.**

6. **Repeat four more times, moving with your breath.**

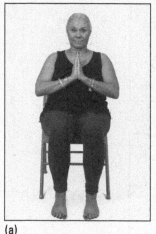 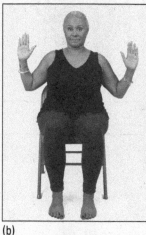 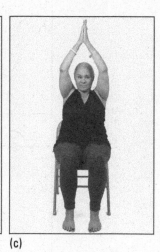

FIGURE 6-4: Wing and a prayer pose.

(a)   (b)   (c)

Shoulder rolls:

1. **Let your arms hang at your sides.**

2. **As you inhale, bring your shoulders up toward your ears and let them draw back (see Figure 6-5).**

3. **As you exhale, bring them back down.**

4. **Repeat three to four more times, moving with your breath.**

5. **Reverse the direction.**

6. **As you inhale, bring your shoulders up toward your ears.**

7. **As you exhale, let them fall forward and all the way back down.**

8. **Repeat three to four more times in this direction, moving with your breath.**

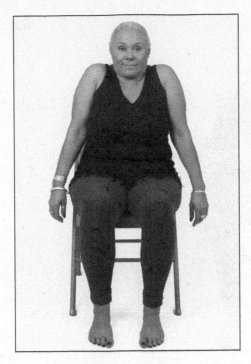

FIGURE 6-5:
Shoulder rolls.

Chair twist:

1. **Sit sideways in your chair.**

2. **Bring your back up tall as you hold on to the back of your chair (see Figure 6-6).**

   Use your inhale to help you sit more upright.

3. **As you exhale, twist toward the back, mainly with your shoulders.**

   Don't over-twist your neck because this step is mainly intended to stretch your back muscles.

   Let each inhalation take you upright, and every exhalation takes you deeper into the twist.

   This twist is intended to relax your muscles and not strain them. Your movements may be slight, even imperceptible. If it hurts at all, don't do it.

4. **Repeat for several smooth breaths and then slowly unwind.**

5. **Turn completely to the other side of the chair and repeat.**

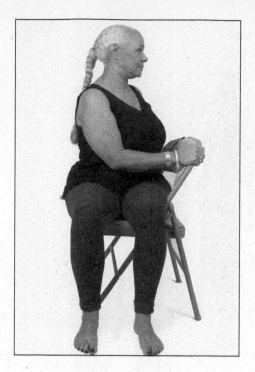

FIGURE 6-6:
Chair twist.

Forward fold using the chair:

1. Slowly come to a standing position and then turn and face the chair.

2. Bring your arms straight out and adjust your distance from the chair so that your extended fingertips hover above the edge of the chair.

3. Bring your arms to your sides.

4. As you inhale, bring your arms straight up over your head.

5. As you exhale, gently bend from your hips, bringing your hands to the chair, allowing your knees to comfortably bend and your head to relax (see Figure 6-7).

6. As you inhale, bring your arms back up, over your head, standing tall.

7. Exhale back down.

8. Keep moving up and down, with your breath, for four more rounds.

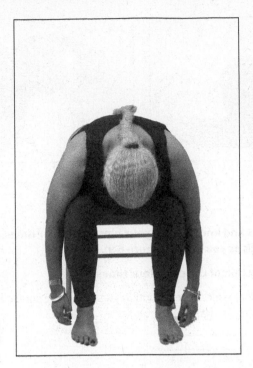

FIGURE 6-7:
Forward fold
using a chair.

Cat/cow is a great routine that continues to lengthen out your spine and warm up your hip and shoulder joints. This pose requires you to come to your hands and knees, so feel free to cushion any place that makes the pose more comfortable — especially your knees.

1. Come to your hands and knees, with the heels of your hands just down from your shoulders and your knees hips-width apart, just under your hips.

2. Bring your arms to your sides.

3. As you inhale, arch your back as you look up.

4. As you exhale, round your back, draw your belly in, and look down (see Figure 6-8).

5. Repeat three more times and then hold in the rounded position with your belly in.

You decide how long to hold this one.

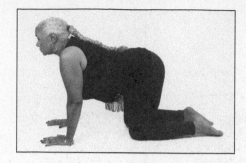

FIGURE 6-8:
Cat/cow.

Hip circles:

1. **From your hands and knees, circle your hips about four times, moving forward and back as you do (see Figure 6-9).**

2. **Reverse the direction of the circle four times.**

TIP

As you circle, explore your range of motion. Again, nothing should hurt. If it does, you're pushing too hard.

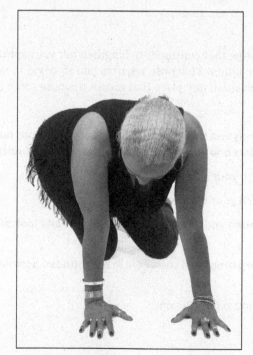

FIGURE 6-9:
Hip circles.

Balancing cat:

1. **As you inhale, slide your right hand forward and your left foot back.**

2. **Lift both of the extended limbs up and out (thumb up on your arm).**

   Ideally, your right hand and left foot are at about the same height (see Figure 6-10). Remember to keep breathing.

3. **Hold this position until you decide when to come down (on an exhalation).**

4. **Repeat on the other side.**

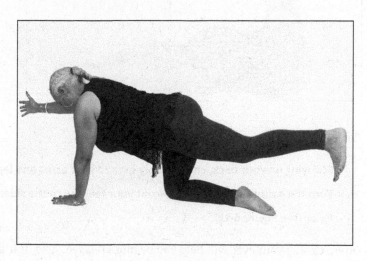

FIGURE 6-10:
Balancing cat.

For the remainder of this 15-minute routine, lie on your mat with your back to the floor.

Supine arms and legs raise:

1. **Bend your knees and place your feet on the ground and your palms face down at your sides.**

2. **Take a deep breath and as you exhale, draw your knees into your chest.**

3. **As you inhale, slowly straighten your legs and bring your arms overhead, ideally touching the ground behind you with your fingertips (see Figure 6-11).**

4. **As you exhale, bend your knees into the chest and bring your arms back down to your sides.**

5. **Repeat four more times.**

TIP

Try to put a definite pause at the top of the movement and at the bottom.

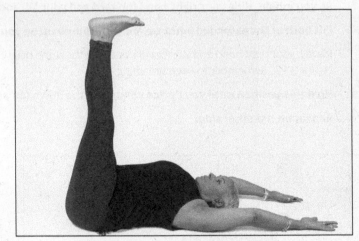

FIGURE 6-11:
Supine arms/
legs raise.

Corpse pose:

1. **Still lying on your back, comfortably extend your arms and legs.**

2. **Turn the palms of your hands up; let your feet fall to the sides.**

3. **Relax (see Figure 6-12).**

TIP

Often, closing your eyes will help you be more relaxed. Also, if it's more comfortable on your spine, feel free to bend your knees.

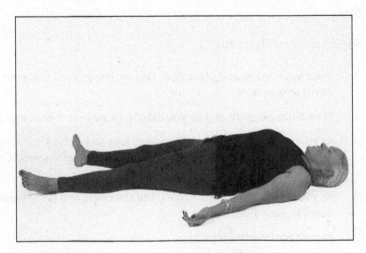

FIGURE 6-12:
Corpse pose.

Five-minute routine

Sometimes your busy life leaves you little time for working out. If you fall into that category, this quick routine is perfect for you. While my hope remains that you find the time to do the 15-minute routine, the shortened version should take you only about 5 minutes.

To complete this routine, simply do the first five poses of the longer routine. These poses are

>> Arm raises

>> Arm raises with head turn

>> Wing and a prayer

>> Shoulder rolls

>> Chair twist

>> Forward fold using a chair

You can get the description of each pose from the full routine listed in the preceding section.

IN THIS CHAPTER

» **Exploring the mind/body connection**

» **Discovering the power of visualization**

» **Making affirmations**

» **Setting goals**

» **Reducing stress through nature, family, and laughter**

Chapter **7**

Connecting Yoga and the Power of the Mind

The practice of Yoga has evolved over at least four centuries, and much of what is taught or emphasized depends upon the particular lineage of the teacher. Yet regardless of the types of Yoga that are taught today, the one aspect they all have in common is that the mind and the body are intricately connected.

The Mind/Body Connection Is Real

Many books are written on the subject of the mind/body connection. While I don't want to give you some kind of history lesson here, I do want to share with you certain characteristics of the mind/body connection that you can apply to improve your everyday life.

Of course, you already know that what's going on in your mind can affect your entire body. If you're in the waiting room at your dentist's office anticipating, say, a root canal procedure, your hands may become sweaty, you feel a bit nauseated, or your neck and back muscles may tighten up. The anticipation, maybe even the fear, that originates somewhere in your mind is now manifesting itself in your physical body. Thoughts can be powerful in that way; you need to learn how to harness that power.

Mind/Body Activities

You may already be doing certain activities that are intended to have positive mental outcomes. Maybe having your morning coffee while watching the news helps you relax and mentally prepare for your day. Other possibly routine activities include:

>> Meditating

>> Praying

>> Listening to or playing music

>> Practicing Tai chi or Qigong

>> Working out

At the top of the list, of course, I recommend Yoga. And while I talk a lot about how physical movement can help make your physical body healthier, it is important to recognize the ways in which Yoga helps you identify what's going on in your mind.

Yoga without the Postures

Practicing Yoga goes far beyond just doing the postures. Yoga is, in fact, an ancient philosophy, and you could argue that the practice provides much more insight on how to live off the Yoga mat than on it.

REMEMBER

The point I want to stress here is that your mind does influence your body. Just as athletes can use the power of their minds to help them excel in their sport, so, too, can you use your mind to help achieve your goals, stay calm, or sometimes even manage chronic pain.

You may have heard the biblical expression "As someone thinks within himself, so he is" (Proverbs 23:7).

Similarly, the Buddha says, "The mind is everything. What you think, you become."

Harvard Medical School published an article in May 2016 titled "How Your Attitudes Affect Your Health." The article talks about how patients' outlook on life and a sense of hope and direction can contribute significantly to positive health outcomes.

I had the privilege of meeting the great Yoga master Swami Satchidananda at the 1994 European Yoga Conference in Switzerland. His words about the power of the mind certainly echo these other great traditions: "There is no limit to the power of the human mind."

Yoga and the Power of Imagination

As a Yoga instructor, I encourage my students to use three practices to use their minds to improve their everyday lives:

» Visualization

» Affirmation

» Goal setting

Visualization

Yoga is more about philosophy than physical poses. One of the goals of Yoga, in the traditional sense, is not just about the postures and movements, but also living life in a way that taps into our inner joy.

Indeed, the early emphasis in Yoga teachings was clearly more cerebral than physical. One way to explore the power of your own mind is through *visualization*. In Yoga, visualization involves creating mental pictures of certain outcomes or qualities, and the ultimate objective is to make those mental images a reality — to bring them into existence.

As a Yoga teacher, I've had the opportunity to work with a lot of professional athletes who use visualization as part of their regular regime. When a basketball player stands at the free throw line, he first imagines what the ball will look like when it drops through the hoop. When a professional golfer lines up a 30-foot putt, she visualizes in her mind what that ball will look like when it rolls up to the cup and drops in. Does it always work? Of course not, but visualization is still a tool used by the pros. And, in both examples, these athletes knew that they already had the talent to succeed.

The power of visualization is a matter of ongoing debate. But science has shown that the mind often perceives the things that are real and the things imagined in the very same way. Centuries of other anecdotal evidence suggests that what you think does, sometimes and in some way, manifest in your life.

I recommend that you try visualization. Here are some tips to guide you:

>> Imagine what attaining a goal will look like or feel like for you.

>> Imagine the emotions you will feel when your visualization becomes a reality.

>> Practice! (You may hear a lifetime of voices in your head telling you why you're wasting your time; don't listen to them and get discouraged.)

>> Share your visualizations with a teacher or someone you trust. Verbally describing your idea of success may cement it better in your mind.

>> Know that you already have everything you need to succeed.

Affirmation

If visualization is a process of imagining what you don't yet have, *affirmation* is a way to acknowledge what you already have. My clients who were professional athletes visualized how they were going to perform on the court or the course, but it was equally important for them to already know that they had the talent, training, and athletic ability to achieve their desired outcome.

And, of course, they had to fight against those old voices telling them otherwise. We all need to ignore some of the old, negative voices. That's what affirmations do. You create new voices — new observations that affirm that you already have what you need to make your dreams come true.

When you create your own affirmation:

>> Be specific.

>> Write it down. You might even want to post it somewhere where you will see it every day — even multiple times a day.

>> Keep it in the present ("I am," not "I will become").

>> Make it succinct (something short and not too complex).

>> Say the affirmation daily.

Goal setting

Visualization, affirmation, and goal setting all interact with one another. Often, people are good about visualizing where they want to go, but not necessarily the steps to get there. By setting specific goals, you can do just that.

Say, for example, a new actor visualizes winning an Academy Award. (I've also had a lot of clients in the entertainment field, and I know firsthand that visualization is often a part of their regime.) Before you can win that award, you probably need to achieve some preliminary goals. Maybe it's attending more acting classes, or auditioning for the movie in the first place. In any case, achieving what you visualize often entails achieving certain goals along the way.

My tips for goal setting?

>> Be specific.

>> Make the goal attainable in the near future (maybe even set a target date for completion).

>> Make the goal something that you can easily measure (even if it's just a checkmark that says, "Did it").

>> Work with a teacher or partner if it helps you to be more accountable.

>> Never doubt that you can achieve your goal; you can even use affirmations to achieve it.

While this entire process is something you can do separately, you can integrate these mental activities within a daily meditation practice. For more information about meditation, see Chapter 5.

Stress as the great saboteur

When I talk about how the mind can affect your body, nothing is more illustrative of this fact than the negative impact of stress. Indeed, stress can manifest itself in

>> Pain (from migraine headaches to backaches)

>> Tight muscles

>> Problems with sleep or sexual function

And stress can lead to unwelcome behaviors, including

>> Eating (overeating, not eating, or other eating disorders)

>> Anti-social or angry behavior

>> Drug and alcohol use

So, reducing or eliminating stress is always a goal — certainly a goal of Yoga.

In Chapter 5, I talk about what it means to be in the moment. Unfortunately, the expression has become a bit trite, even in the Yoga community. Yet the only thing you are trying to accomplish by being in the moment is simply to not let your mind dwell on things that have already happened or on things yet to happen. Instead, focus solely on the here and now — the present.

I'd like to highlight here three different approaches that can help keep you in the present moment to avoid stress:

>> Spending time in nature

>> Spending time with family

>> Laughing

Spending time in nature

While it's certainly possible to be present while standing in line at the supermarket or inching along in bumper-to-bumper traffic, the outdoors has a way of bringing people completely into the moment and even keeping them there.

Maybe it's the majesty of it, the sheer beauty of it, or the wonderful overload of the senses with her sights and sounds, smells, and textures. Without a doubt, regardless of the reasons, your stress will likely begin to dissipate when you immerse yourself in nature. Why do you think most Yoga retreats are in beautiful locations?

REMEMBER

And, as a practical matter, you don't need the Grand Canyon to experience the benefits of being in the outdoors. Try a daily walk on a nearby hiking trail or even around the yard or neighborhood; it can do wonders.

Spending time with your family

Humans, by nature, need companionship. Recent studies conducted by Harvard University and New York University, among other places, explore the correlation between social relationships and medical outcomes. Loneliness, it turns out, is as bad for your health as obesity and smoking.

If you happen to be lucky enough to have family members near you, spending time in their company may be good for your mind and your body.

I know, of course, that families can also be the cause of stress. From the demands of day-to-day life to finances, sickness, divorce, and death— all these things may have a negative impact on everyone involved. And, just maybe, you're the only one who can start to mend things. If so, give it a try.

But maybe your family life is all good. And I'm sure I don't have to tell you how wonderful it feels to put your arm around your mom, give your child a hug, or maybe even bounce your grandchild on your knee. You can almost feel the rush of endorphins (those feel-good hormones) flowing through your body.

The reality, however, is we all get busy. Sometimes, you have to make the effort to keep your connections with family and friends alive and thriving. Do it! It's always worth it.

Laughing

I hope you're not looking for a good joke in this section. The beauty is when you start laughing, the body doesn't really know whether it's a real laugh or you're just pretending. In fact, that's the idea behind Laughing Yoga, which is a worldwide movement.

Laughing is infectious, and scattered outbursts of fake laughter usually evolve into a roomful of the real thing. Certainly enough studies have concluded that laughter increases the production of endorphins and reduces the production of cortisol (the stress hormone).

So, how is laughing good for you? It has great power to

>> Decrease stress

>> Decrease pain

>> Reduce anxiety

» Boost immunity

» Relax tight muscles

» Promote a healthy heart

» Put you in a better mood

If you find something that you watch or read that makes you laugh, or maybe you have a comedy club nearby, by all means enjoy the benefits that come from true laughter. But if real laughs are not so accessible, you should definitely try pretending; see what it feels like to smile and then laugh out loud. You can still get all the health benefits, and your body won't really know the difference. (And I'll never tell!)

IN THIS CHAPTER

» **Reaping the benefits of a good night's sleep**

» **Blocking out blue light**

» **Trying Yogic sleep**

» **Remembering your Vitamin G**

» **Practicing at home to manage sleep**

» **Finding a Yogic approach to greater intimacy**

Chapter **8**

Bedtime Yoga

When considering your overall health, getting a good night's sleep is critical. Yet too many people struggle with falling asleep or getting back to sleep after waking up in the middle of the night. In this chapter, I share with you some of the ways that Yoga can help.

At the heart of Yoga is the recognition of the mind/body connection, so some of the following sleep routines target what's going on in your head — what's on your mind (see Chapter 7 for more about the mind/body connection). If you can steady your mind, your body will likely follow suit — and that is as much a Yoga practice as doing a downward-facing dog on your mat.

Your Mind and Sleep

We all know that sleep is beneficial to our mind and bodies, and that sleep deprivation can lead to a multitude of harmful effects. For certain people, falling and staying asleep is not an issue at all; for others, bedtime can be something to dread.

The reality is that if you're having problems falling or staying asleep, it may have more to do with what's going on in your mind than in your body. Oftentimes, it's stress that keeps you awake — and stress can stem from countless things going on in your life.

While I can't promise you that a good night's sleep will change everything, enough research suggests that sleep, preceded by a reduction of stress, can have a positive impact in any one of the following areas:

>> Anxiety

>> Depression

>> Inflammations in the body

>> Longevity

>> Memory

>> Creativity/problem solving

>> Attentiveness/focus

>> Weight management

The relationship between stress and all these areas is the subject of ongoing study. What seems to be true, however, is that when you're stressed, the brain attempts to come to your aid by signaling the production of hormones, such as cortisol or adrenaline. These chemicals can be a great help if you're going into battle or perhaps running away from it. If, however, your only goal is to fall asleep, these stimulating hormones won't be helpful at all.

That's why reducing stress and the production of certain hormones associated with stress can have an array of positive effects. This, for example, probably explains why people who start a meditation regime often experience unanticipated weight loss. (For more on this topic, see Chapter 6.)

Yoga and Sleep

So, how specifically does Yoga address sleep issues? Centuries of anecdotal evidence (or at least decades of anecdotal evidence that I personally picked up from my students and patients) points to a number of important ways Yoga can help:

>> A physical practice (like other forms of exercise) can simply make you more tired and more likely to fall asleep.

>> Yoga can help reduce the impact of stress and anxiety (which then makes it easier to fall and stay asleep).

>> Yoga brings a sense of calm and safety, both of which are particularly conducive to sleep.

Blue light versus Yoga

One of the challenges today that the ancient Yogis didn't have to deal with is *blue light* — that ghastly glow emanating from various electronic devices that people bathe themselves in before bed.

Blue light itself may not be particularly harmful. It's all that blue light just before bed that becomes the problem. In the old days, before electricity, bodies knew the difference between night and day based on the rising and setting of the sun. Once artificial light came into use, the time of day became much more difficult to assess, and the internal body clock —your *circadian rhythm* — suddenly became more compromised.

While the disruption of the circadian rhythm may not be a new challenge to sleep, the recent proliferation of electronic devices has compounded the problem thoroughly. The body is designed to produce melatonin at night to help you sleep. When you immerse your brain in blue light, your body doesn't know that it's night time and doesn't produce that sleep-inducing melatonin.

TIP

So, how do you handle it? The general rule is to stop gazing at electronic devices for two to three hours prior to going to bed. I wish I had some Yoga magic that would help you with this one, but I don't. You just have to turn off your gadgets.

You could always designate this prebedtime period for your home Yoga routine. People who like to work out late at night may find this strategy workable, but others may not.

Rose-colored glasses

Some sleep experts say that wearing blue-light-filtering glasses — though typically amber, not rose-colored — will protect you from sleep-disrupting blue light. I'm sure, of course, that this approach will continue to be the subject of many studies. In the meantime, you may want to try the glasses, particularly when avoiding screens two to three hours before bed seems like an unrealistic objective.

Not surprisingly, there are also apps that do the same thing. Ranging in price from free to a modest fee, these smartphone apps are designed to filter out blue light. This, I suspect, may be better for you than staring at your phone at night when it's unfiltered, but these apps are new and still improving.

Don't Forget Your Vitamin G

If stress is the enemy of sleep, then gratitude may be its greatest ally. Gratitude — or *Vitamin G*, as some people call it — is being recognized, even by mainstream Western medicine, as a powerful tool in managing stress, depression, the rate of healing, and even pain.

Indeed, if you want to set your mind on a gentler path before trying to sleep, consider making a conscious effort to identify things for which you're grateful. You could do this by merely taking time to reflect on your life or even be more formal and start a gratitude journal — some kind of journal or notebook by your bedside. Each night before closing your eyes, you write, or say, three things you are grateful for. Bringing your focus on these things, whether it's family, health, or even your comfy bed, can help relieve stress, induce relaxation, and make you more susceptible to falling asleep.

TIP

Being specific will make your Vitamin G much more powerful.

Things to Think About

If sleeping is not something that comes easy to you, it is important to recognize that you have a problem that may not only impact you emotionally, but can also have negative health consequences. So, take the following suggestions to heart:

>> Establish and stick to a set routine for going to bed.

>> Make sure your day contains some physical activity or exercise to help make you more tired at bedtime (personally, I recommend Yoga!).

>> Avoid taking naps during the day (and yes, I know this can be challenging if you're not sleeping at night).

>> Avoid that dreaded blue light several hours before bedtime (see the section earlier in this chapter).

>> Find something positive to think about that will keep your steer your mind away from stressful topics.

>> Don't watch the clock.

>> Don't bring relationship issues to bed (mend the probler anyone in your life).

>> Don't try to force sleep (take comfort in knowing that by just lying in bed, your body is getting the rest it needs).

Yoga Sleep

Sometimes referred to as *Yoga Nidra, Yoga sleep* describes a state in which the body completely relaxes, while the mind remains at least somewhat focused.

The practice is as old as Yoga itself and is sometimes viewed as a form of meditation. It is actually quite different, however. During meditation, your mind stays on a conscious level. You certainly attempt to change that conscious state, to allow for more steadiness or focus, but that all happens on a relatively conscious level.

Yoga sleep attempts to bring you gradually to your subconscious mind — the place where all your old torments reside, all the thoughts and feelings that prevent you from sleeping. In simple terms, using Yoga sleep, you try to replace those old torments with newer, more positive resolutions.

TIP

You may want to think of Yoga Nidra more as an alternative to sleep, rather than a pathway to it. Using this technique, practitioners often find they derive the same benefits as they do from a good night's sleep. Other people find that the practice itself actually helps them fall asleep.

Either way, Yoga Nidra can be a powerful tool for dealing with both sleep disorders and stress. Many books have been written on the subject, and Dr. Richard Miller, a dear friend and colleague, has done some pioneering work using Yoga Nidra techniques to address post-traumatic stress disorder (PTSD) issues with returning veterans. (His version is called Integrative Rest, or iRest.)

Note: Richard Miller is a world-renowned Yogic teacher, author, scholar, and researcher, as well as a clinical psychologist. In addition to creating iRest, which has offered profound benefits to many, including soldiers returning from Iraq and Afghanistan suffering from PTSD, Richard is also cofounder, with me, of the International Association of Yoga Therapists. You can read more about Richard at www.irest.org.

Yoga sleep scripts

One of the essential components of a Yoga Nidra session is the *guide* — the voice of the person leading you into a conscious state of deep relaxation. Practicing at home can be problematic if you expect to have a live person sitting at the foot of your bed, leading your session. But lying back and listening to a recording (to someone whose voice you like and whose words are soothing) is easy enough (see Figure 8-1).

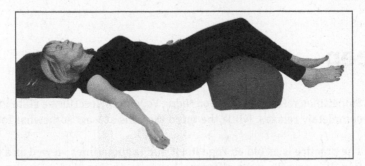

FIGURE 8-1: Relaxing for a Yoga Nidra session.

You can find recordings to purchase that may help you experience a Yoga sleep session at home.

These recordings are also available (some at no charge) on some of the meditation apps, including

- >> Calm
- >> Headspace
- >> Insight Timer

Developing an intention or resolve

Yoga sleep will attempt to bring you into your subconscious mind — to help you get beneath the surface. When you get there, you want to bring with it an intention, or resolve, regarding yourself and your life. Typically, you should select something that doesn't involve economic gain, though common examples often include finding personal or professional success. Other intentions might focus on personal health or the health of those around you. You may also create a resolve to be a positive presence in someone's life.

This intention will then be used to supplant certain detrimental thought patterns that have no basis in your present reality, that may in fact be the residue of another time (like childhood), that may be a leading cause of the stress in your life (especially bedtime stress), and that is actually helping to shape the general flow of your life — for the worse.

The new resolve, then, is an essential part of Yoga sleep. That's why I hope you will give it some thought; the more powerful your resolve or intention, the more effective the Yoga Nidra practice will be.

The following tips may come in handy when creating your own intention:

>> Make it succinct and easy to state.

>> Choose wording you can remember and repeat.

>> Identify an intention or resolve that will bring about a positive change in you or in your life.

>> Remember that you are bringing this thought into your subconscious.

I coming up with your own resolve actually creates more stress for you, let it go. You don't have to come up with the perfect intention right from the start. In fact, maybe the process itself — the trips back and forth into your subconscious mind — will reveal some of the sources of your stress and bring to mind a new declaration that will ultimately serve you better. In this case, patience could indeed be a virtue.

Yoga Sleep at Home

I've created a home practice for you that can be a good place to start if you're considering further exploration of Yoga Nidra. In this exercise, you will achieve focus, not by listening to someone else, but rather by directing your mind to perform what is sometimes called a *body scan*.

1. **Lie flat on your back, with your arms in a comfortable position.**

TIP

   If needed, place a pillow or folded blanket behind your neck for support and another pillow or folded blanket under your knees for added comfort (see Figure 8-2).

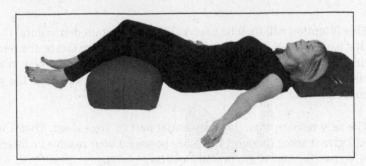

FIGURE 8-2:
Yoga Nidra
position.

2. **Let your eyes gently close.**

3. **Take some deep breaths, breathing only through the nose (if possible).**

4. **Visualize your entire body lying comfortably on the floor (this is called *Whole Body Awareness*).**

5. **Bring to mind a resolve, or intention, or course of action.**

6. **Starting with the right side of your body, let your mental awareness scan that side of your body (in the following sequence):**

   - Right thumb, index, middle, ring, and little finger

   - Palm of the hand

   - Back of the hand

   - Wrist

   - The right hand as a whole

   - Forearm

   - Elbow

   - Upper arm

   - Shoulder joint

   - Shoulder

   - Neck

   - The face (forehead, eyes, nose, mouth, chin)

   - Right ear

   - Scalp

   - Throat

   - Chest

   - Side of the rib cage

- Right shoulder blade
- Waist
- Stomach
- Lower abdomen
- Genitals
- Thigh
- The right knee
- Shin
- Calf
- Ankle
- Top of the right foot
- Heel
- Sole
- Big toe and remaining toes

7. **Be aware of your body as a whole.**

8. **Repeat the scan in Step 6 on the left side of your body, again ending with the whole-body awareness.**

9. **Next, visualize the back side of your body:**
- How the back of your head touches the floor or neck support
- Right and left shoulders
- Upper back
- Hips
- Back of your thighs
- Calves
- Heels

10. **Again, focus on your intention and finish with overall body awareness again (like in Step 4).**

You can drift off to sleep now. If you're getting up, roll to one side and push up; don't start by lifting your head forward.

TIP

You're not constrained by time in this exercise, so take as much or as little time as you need. The tempo is up to you.

This particular routine does not require you to follow a recording, but instead requires you to focus on the body scan process. And please don't think you have to memorize or keep coming back to the preceding list. My only intention is to give you a sense of where to start and end and some points you may want to hit along the way. Don't worry if you leave out body parts or even add parts I don't have on the list.

Yoga and Intimate Matters

When it comes to intimacy, the focus is often on the physical. But, just like with Yoga, there are other critical aspects to consider. Learning how to better communicate with a partner, for example, can deepen the overall experience and strengthen your intimate relationships.

Of course, there are specific aspects of intimacy to keep in mind as you age. Unfortunately, it seems that culture tends to depict romantic relationships in the earlier stages of life. But I would like to suggest to you that, despite what you see on TV or in movies, intimate relationships later in life can be even more fulfilling.

How yoga can support intimacy in physical expressions

Movies, music, and ads sell us all day long on how being that virile 20-something is what's key — always with a product, procedure, or potion in mind. And then we risk a look in the mirror and think, "Woe is me!" The reality is our bodies, performance, mobility, and appearance change across time. And that's okay. In fact, it's natural. Plus, there are so many positive sides of being our age: We're better at problem solving, less worried about what others think, generally more happy, care more about other people, and much more.

What would our marketplaces look like if we stressed the positive aspects of aging? It would look very different, indeed. But that doesn't mean that Yoga doesn't offer benefits when it comes to looking or feeling younger. It's just that striving to deny the normal aging process shouldn't be our focus.

Yoga and sex

An active sex life requires poses, flexibility, and capacities that are much like a Yoga practice. But just as you modify your Yoga poses and movements, you also need to understand and communicate with your partner so that you both can adapt to changes such as a stiff hip, worn wrist, or cardiac limitation.

MARKETING MISSES THE MARK

I started out in the advertising and marketing field before my Yoga career — and my generation certainly knows marketing!

Anyone remember *The Pepsi Generation* campaign? Of course you do. That term sums up what drives so much of western marketing. Stay young, trim, tight skinned, and wrinkle-free and perform like a hormone-rich teenager!

This campaign of dissatisfaction if you aren't that way is an unconscious, highly imaged dominant mind trap that we're all stuck in. Think about it. You never hear "Highlight those hard-earned wrinkles or accent that receding hairline." No, the marketing hook, the quest, is to stay young, perform young.

How does Yoga look at *marketing* growing older? Very differently.

In Yoga, aging is a natural and rewarding process, each phase with its proper emphasis. Yoga describes three distinct life phases:

- Early years of growth and discovery to include finding life purpose/vocation and relationships

- A period of working hard, growing businesses/families

- A well-earned period of slowing down to savor and gather the wisdom of experience, as well as to deeply examine who we really are and what is most important in life

Many of us are in that second or third phase right now. And the Yoga campaign seems much healthier than the other, doesn't it?

TIP

Let your partner see into who you are today and trust that the insight will deepen the intimacy (in-to-see-me) with someone who truly cares about you. Feeling the freedom to share the same things back with you is healthy and Yogic — especially compared to suffering quietly, or just plain avoiding certain activities without explanation.

Also, in the same way I address nutrition and suggest seeking out a nutritionist for support, you should do the same thing for any physical limitations. Is there rehabilitation for that stiff hip of yours? Can you modify a position to support your well-worn wrist? The answer is probably, so seek out support. Don't just deny your problem.

Communicating openly and then slowing things down, to savor and linger (versus blasting through), is the benefit of this wisdom phase and should not be a source of embarrassment or sense of failure. Is it easy to talk about? No. Is it important to stay steady and calm in intimacy? Absolutely.

So, just as you need to ask yourself or your teacher for trust and guidance in Yoga poses, you also need to ask for the same trust and guidance from your partner. In being vulnerable, you can deepen your intimacy and strengthen your relationship. You get all this by just being your age.

Professionals can support and guide you if initiating this line of communication with your partner is too big a stretch to do on your own. Seek out the support you might need.

Yoga and optimal pelvic floor health

Doing the Yoga practices in this book can optimize your reproductive health and the function of the critical muscles of the pelvic floor. The science is in. Many of the problems related to function and performance over 50 are not so natural as just being the result of our overstressed, inactive lifestyles.

When you begin to move safely, in wider ranges of motion, under control and then deeply relaxed, it improves reproductive health. Again, specialists, both Yoga therapists and other health professionals, can give fuller support when you identify your challenges. Do that awkward pose of seeking them out and maximize your opportunities for deeper intimacy.

Yoga after medical procedures

The consequences of certain medical procedures can either directly or indirectly affect intimacy. And they happen. A lot. A short list includes

>> Hysterectomy and related procedures

>> Prostatectomy, orchiectomy, and variants

>> Repair of childbirth trauma of the pelvic floor

>> Mastectomy, breast reconstruction, and other scarring procedures

>> Hernias, bladder reconstructions, uterine prolapse, bowel repair, and other lower abdomen surgeries

So, what does Yoga have to say about all these potential obstacles to your intimate relationship?

First, you can talk about the effect of the procedure and understand more deeply what the other person is going through, while communicating your needs in an objective, non-critical way. If you can't or don't want to do that, would you be willing to seek out professional support with a highly trained sex therapist? For pelvic health for women and men, there is an entire specialty section in physical therapy you can tap into.

Again, communication might feel awkward. But having the wisdom to look deeply at these issues is what this phase of life in Yoga is all about.

Celebrating what we share

Your single Yoga pose in this chapter is to reflect on what applies to you and your partner. Then, can you make that reflection a celebration of the changes in life despite what the dominant marketing suggests?

REMEMBER

Slow down. Sense what each of you need. Talk to each other about what each of you needs. Modify your positions and use props when you need to. Be patient. Savor these fleeting minutes together. Hug just a bit tighter and longer.

None of us gets out of here alive — and only some of us ever get to celebrate this adventure, deeply, with another special person.

REMEMBER

In the world of Yoga, intimacy is about deepening the connection — and communication.

4

Adapting Your Practice to Common 50-Plus Conditions

IN THIS PART . . .

Learn how Yoga can help you with balance.

Identify Yoga approaches to accommodate back, knee, and other conditions.

Review home Yoga practices designed to accommodate or help prevent certain conditions.

Chapter **9**

Keeping Your Balance

One of the first things you did when you came into this world is deal with the challenge of finding your balance. While your memories may be a bit hazy on this formidable journey, you've perhaps watched a baby first learning to crawl, then taking its first step or two, and finally learning to walk.

You may have a better recollection of exactly what it took for you to ride a bicycle. There may have been a lot falling, a lot of tears — maybe even some training wheels. Do you remember thinking, "It's just never going to happen"? But then one day, miraculously, it did. And as you cruised around the neighborhood on just two wheels, you may have made a fleeting observation that, in the end, it was pretty easy.

The good news — is that, with practice and determination, the brain and body discover how to find balance. And that fact doesn't change as we get older.

What does change with age is your resiliency. And what that means to you during physical activity is pretty straightforward:

» You are more prone to injury.

» Injuries may be more serious and probably will have a greater impact.

» Injuries will take longer to heal.

In fact, falls are the leading cause of both fatal and nonfatal injuries to older Americans.

Knowing this should be a huge incentive for you to make sure that you're giving adequate attention to your ability to maintain balance.

Proprioception: The Key to All Yoga Poses

A scientific term that is *proprioception*. Your proprioception relates directly to your ability to balance.

Proprioception simply refers to your ability to know where your body is in space. So, whether you're walking along a sidewalk at night, descending a dark set of stairs, or even doing a Yoga pose, your brain, with the help of various proprioceptors throughout your body, tries to determine exactly how your body is moving and what position your limbs are in at any given moment.

I've always been fascinated by the proprioception that cats have. Ever watch them fall from a high place and land on all fours, calm and unhurt? Or, ever observe them balance on a very narrow surface and never wobble? Pretty amazing!

When it comes to human balance, your ankles and feet provide a lot of this feedback because they are working so hard to keep you from falling. It's important, then, to give these areas some attention first by warming them up.

Warmups may include:

>> Taking your body weight off of these structures (lying on your mat, for example, with your legs in the air)

>> Pointing and flexing your feet

>> Rotating your ankles one way and then the other

>> Spreading and crunching your toes

Each of these movements will either stretch muscles or help lubricate your joints. And by adding the standing balance poses that I introduce in this chapter, these movements will better prepare you to strengthen the muscles and ligaments around your ankles and feet.

Practicing Poses: Pointers to Keep in Mind

REMEMBER

Balance improves with practice (at any age), so practice. Again, the stakes get higher the older you get.

Of course, you should never lose sight of the fact that wobbling and catching yourself as you fall out of a pose is all part of the process. You may feel that losing your balance is like losing the game, but you couldn't be more mistaken. Every wobble is information that your brain uses to recalibrate, information that will help you the next time you try to balance. And like first learning to walk or riding a bike, you'll get better with practice.

Practice up against the wall

You can practice many of the balancing poses with your hand or hands on a wall, which can be helpful if falling over is a real possibility. You can always take your hand away if you want to practice without support — in fact, maybe it's good enough to just have a wall or post close by (just in case).

I often use props in Yoga. Props can help you get deeper into a pose, get into a pose more safely, and hold a pose in a way that is beneficial. Sometimes, knowing when to use a prop is a true sign of advanced Yoga (regardless of how traditionally perfect it looks). A wall can be a great assistant.

Keep your eyes steady

In addition to ankles and toes, you should also think about your eyes — or, more specifically, what you are looking at.

TIP

When you're doing a pose that challenges your balance, try fixing your eyes on something stationary. If you're watching something that's moving around — maybe outside your window or perhaps an energetic Yoga teacher in the front of the room — finding your balance can prove even more difficult. Before you move into a balance pose, fix your gaze on a spot on the wall or a crack in the floor. Keeping your eyes steady will help you keep your entire body steady.

And if you're at all in doubt about how much what you're looking at relates to your ability to balance, try doing any balance pose with your eyes closed. If you try this exercise, make sure someone is standing close by to spot you because you will definitely start to fall.

Remember breathing is everything

My last bit of advice before introducing the most basic balancing postures is to always remember to breathe. While I talk about the breath in more detail in Chapter 3, maintaining an even breathing pattern is important to holding your balance.

In Yoga, the more precarious a movement or posture may be, the more your breathing pattern is affected. And what's more precarious than being in a balancing pose, feeling like you're going to fall at any moment?

Your instinct may be to hold your breath, a signal to you from your brain that you may be in trouble. When that happens, you respond in ways that cause tension — both emotional and physical — as your system prepares you to possibly hit the ground.

TIP

Instead of sending that signal, make sure you keep breathing. If standing near a wall, maybe even touching it, makes it easier to breathe, then do it. You didn't learn to walk without a lot of practice; you didn't learn to ride a bike without a lot of practice. The Yoga mat is not the place to suddenly lose patience. Keep breathing; balance and confidence will eventually come.

Alignment and Balancing Poses

In the following sections, I cover postures that will challenge your sense of balance:

>> Balancing cat

>> Karate Kid

>> Tree

>> Warrior III at the wall

Balancing cat

Balancing cat, shown in Figure 9-1, is great for working on your balance because you are near to the ground. Also, you will feel your core muscles engage as you try to maintain your balance, which makes this pose one of the best for abdominal strengthening.

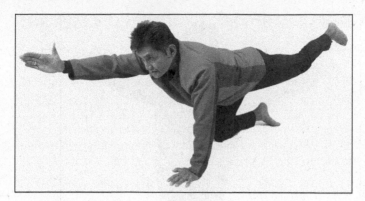

FIGURE 9-1:
Balancing cat
pose.

To get into this pose:

1. Beginning on your hands and knees, position your hands directly under your shoulders with your palms down, your fingers spread on the floor, and your knees directly under your hips.

2. Straighten your arms, but don't lock your elbows.

3. As you exhale, slide your right hand forward and your left leg back, keeping your left hand and right toes on the floor.

4. As you inhale, raise your left arm and right leg to a comfortable height, as Figure 9-1 illustrates.

5. Stay in Step 3 for six to eight breaths and then repeat Steps 1 through 3 with opposite pairs (right arm and left leg).

To modify the pose to make it more accessible:

» As you start to extend your arm and opposite leg, keep your hand and foot on the ground first; then lift off the ground, one at a time.

» Just extend your arm and keep both knees on the ground.

Karate kid

This standing pose, known as Karate kid, develops your overall balance while it strengthens the legs, arms, and hips — all parts of the rest of the body that help support your ankles (see Figure 9-2).

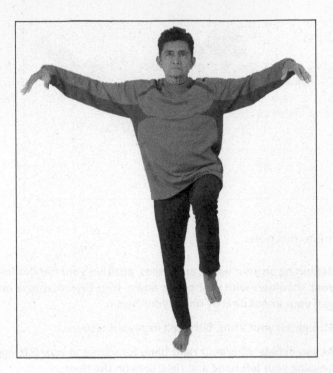

FIGURE 9-2:
Karate kid pose.

To get into this pose, stand upright on your mat:

REMEMBER

1. **As you inhale, raise your arms out to the sides parallel to the line of your shoulders (and the floor) so that they form a T with your torso.**

   To steady yourself, focus on a spot on the floor 10 to 12 feet in front of you.

2. **As you exhale, bend your left knee, raising it toward your chest, while keeping your right leg straight.**

3. **Remain in this posture for six to eight breaths.**

4. **Repeat this sequence using the right knee.**

To modify the pose to make it more accessible:

» Stand near a wall so that you can use it for support. You can touch the wall with one hand. Remember, you can always take your hand off the wall as your balance improves.

» Keep your knee directly in front of you and don't worry about how high you can lift it. The primary purpose of this pose is just to work on your balance.

Tree

When you see Yogis on magazine covers or perhaps on social media posts, it seems like the pose most often chosen is the tree pose. It's a classic balance posture that works your muscles and joints from your ankle and foot all the way up to your arms and shoulders (see Figure 9-3).

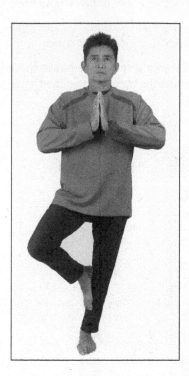

FIGURE 9-3:
Tree pose.

To get into this pose, stand upright on your mat:

1. **As you exhale, bend your right knee and place the sole of your right foot, toes pointing down, on the inside of your left leg, between your knee and your groin.**

2. **As you inhale, bring your arms over your head and join your palms together.**

3. **Soften your arms and focus on a spot 6 to 8 feet in front of you on the floor as shown in Figure 9-3.**

4. **Stay for 6 to 8 breaths.**

5. **Repeat with the other leg.**

To modify the pose to make it more accessible:

>> Don't hesitate to practice this pose near a wall — even if you choose not to use it.

>> Lower the foot on your upper thigh to the inside of your calf, just below your knee. It's best to rest your foot either above or below your knee joint, but not right on it.

>> Hands can even be on your hips if that helps you balance.

>> If having your foot anywhere on your inner leg seems too challenging, you can use the *kickstand* technique where the big toe of the lifted leg can actually be on the ground (see Figure 9-4).

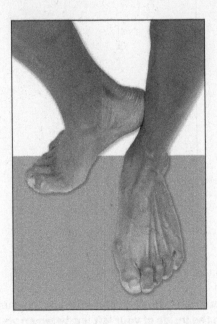

FIGURE 9-4:
Kickstand
technique.

Warrior III at the wall

This variation of the classic warrior III pose challenges your body to stretch and hold while demanding a lot of focus to retain your balance.

To get into this pose:

1. **Stand on your mat, facing a blank wall (about 3 feet away).**

2. **As you exhale, bend forward from the hips and extend your arms forward until your fingertips are touching the wall.**

Adjust yourself so that your legs are perpendicular and your torso and arms are parallel with the floor.

3. **As you inhale, raise your left leg back and up until it's parallel to the floor (see Figure 9-5).**

4. **Stay in Step 3 for six to eight breaths.**

5. **Repeat this sequence with the right leg.**

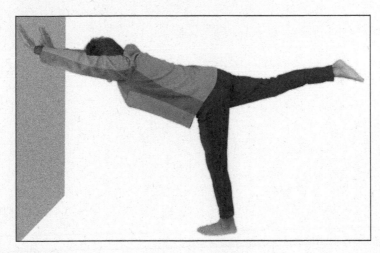

FIGURE 9-5:
Warrior III
at the wall.

To modify the pose to make it more accessible:

>> Warrior III is traditionally done without the wall, so the preceding steps are already making the pose more accessible.

>> Remember the concept of forgiving limbs (I introduce the idea in Chapter 4). Feel free to bend your supporting leg and extended arms, softening them just enough to make the pose more comfortable.

Chapter **10**

Love Your Lower Back

L ower back pain is a condition that almost everyone will experience, sooner or later. In fact, if you're over 50 and you still haven't had to deal with pain in your lower back, you have my congratulations.

Back Pain Is a Common Problem

The statistics relating to back pain are sobering:

» Four out of every five Americans will seek professional help for a back problem sometime in their life.

» Lower back pain is the single leading cause of disability worldwide.

» Back pain is one of the most common reasons for missed work — in fact, back pain is the second most common reason for visits to the doctor's office, outnumbered only by upper respiratory infections.

» Most cases of back pain are mechanical or non-organic, which means they are not caused by serious conditions, such as inflammatory arthritis, infection, fracture, or cancer.

» Americans spend billions of dollars each year treating back pain (and that's just for the more easily identified costs).

It was, in fact, my own lower back pain many years ago that originally brought me to a Yoga class and ultimately set me on a very Yoga-focused life journey. Through the guidance of experienced doctors and Yoga teachers, as well as my own personal dedication and persistence, I found Yoga to be extremely helpful in relieving and ultimately resolving my own back issues.

As a Yoga therapist who specializes in dealing with back issues, I believe that the most common cause of lower back pain is lack of activity (including poor sitting or prolonged sitting). Indeed, some experts claim that sitting is now the new smoking, though the degree to which sitting can negatively impact your health is still a matter of debate.

Nonetheless, the lack of activity is currently seen as contributing to

>> Excessive weight gain

>> Lower back and neck pain

>> Certain types of cancers linked to inactivity

>> Heart disease and diabetes

REMEMBER

This Yoga book or even your own personal practice is not intended to take the place of your doctor. I see Yoga interventions as being more complementary in nature rather than alternative therapy. That idea is particularly true for back pain because it can have so many different causes.

So, before you go any further, if you're in acute pain, you should talk to your doctor. Your treatment options will vary based on your diagnosis, and that diagnosis will also shape your Yoga practice.

It Hurts When I Bend Forward

I refer to movements such as bending forward or rounding your back that causes you pain as *flexion faults*. Symptoms of flexion faults include:

>> Pain when bending forward

>> Pain that's triggered by or made worse from sitting

>> Pain when you do certain Yoga poses that require you to fold (for example, a standing or seated forward bend can be the cause of excruciating pain for people who have trouble rounding their spine)

It is so important for you to let your doctor try to figure out what's wrong with your back if you're in pain. Do not expect your Yoga teacher or even a Yoga therapist to make that diagnosis. Even with the advantages of being able to order X-rays or MRIs, doctors often have a hard time diagnosing the problem.

Having said that, the most common causes of flexion faults tend to be

- ❯❯ Strained muscles (also referred to as strained/sprained, pulled, or spasmed muscles)
- ❯❯ Disc problems (herniated, bulging, or protruding discs)
- ❯❯ Sacroiliac irritation
- ❯❯ Most sciaticas

Yoga postures to avoid

WARNING

If you have been diagnosed with any of the conditions associated with flexion faults, you should avoid Yoga poses that require you to bend or round your back.

Yoga postures that may bring relief

So many of the Yoga postures hightlighted in this book allow for a slight arching of the back, which may feel good. (It moves your spine in the opposite direction of that painful rounding.)

In certain poses, arching (or extending) your back is at the heart of the posture. These poses include the poses in the cobra family for stretching (see Figure 10-1), and the locust family for strengthening (see Figure 10-2).

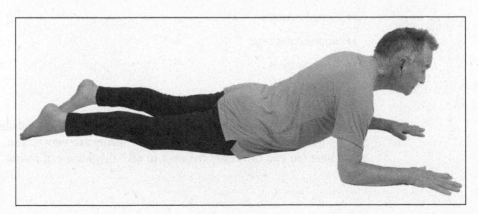

FIGURE 10-1: Cobra pose example.

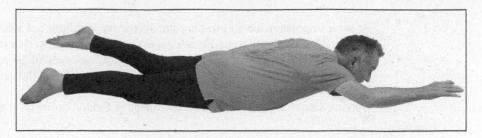

FIGURE 10-2:
Locust pose
example.

It Hurts When I Bend Backwards

Certain back conditions allow a person to bend forward with no discomfort at all, but bending backwards is painful. I refer to that type of pain as an *extension fault*.

Symptoms of extension faults are:

>> Pain when bending backwards

>> Relief when bending forward

>> Pain when doing certain Yoga postures that require you to arch your back (even doing a simple cobra pose with arms in sphinx position can trigger pain)

WARNING

Just like with pain from bending forward, if your back hurts when you bend backwards, you should talk to your doctor about it. Knowing exactly what's causing the pain will help with your strategy for dealing with it. Your Yoga teacher should not be offering a diagnosis or treatment.

From my experience, the most common causes of extension faults are:

>> Facet syndromes

>> Spinal stenosis

>> Spondylolisthesis

>> Spondylolysis

>> Pregnancy

If you've been diagnosed with any of these conditions, you probably know exactly what's going on inside your body. If these terms are new to you, I don't explain them here (so you can resist the urge to self-diagnose). Of course, there is plenty of information available to you on all of these conditions, so you're encouraged to explore further if you're so inclined.

Yoga postures to avoid

If you're dealing with pain from bending backwards, avoid any of the back bending poses, such as those in the cobra family or the locust family. Even lying on your mat with your legs stretched out below you causes your spine to arch a bit, so it may be more comfortable to bend your knees while lying down.

Also, keep your back flat in all your Yoga poses. You may need to bend forward slightly to stay out of pain, but at least your body can benefit from the poses.

For example, by bending slightly forward while doing a warrior I pose, the pain from arching your back will disappear, and you'll be able to stay in the pose, which strengthens the upper thigh of the forward leg and stretches the hamstring of the leg in the back (see Figure 10-3).

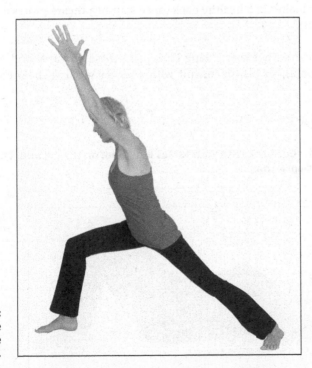

FIGURE 10-3:
Warrior I while bending the spine.

Yoga postures that may bring relief

If bending backward causes you pain, the poses that bend you forward may provide relief. These poses include:

» Standing forward folds

» Seated forward folds

» Knees to chest

» Abdominal exercises

At-Home Routine

The following routine basically contains the same sequence that I recently provided to a major medical school. The poses in this sequence are typically good for helping to maintain a healthy back (once your healthcare professional says you're ready for it).

WARNING

If you're currently experiencing back pain, these postures and movements may not be helpful, so please consult with your doctor first, before attempting this sequence.

Attunement:

1. **Lie on your back with your knees bent, feet on the ground, and palms up (see Figure 10-4).**

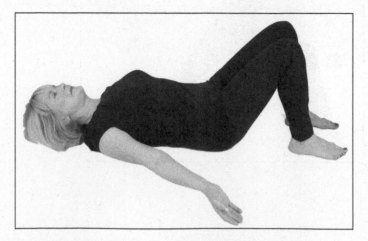

FIGURE 10-4: Attunement.

TIP

2. **Breathe in and out through the nose six to eight times.**

   Try to be in the moment, linking your body, breath, and mind. Use this link to your breath in all postures.

Knee to chest:

1. **Lie on your back with both legs straight.**

2. **As you exhale, draw your right knee into your chest and bring the toes of your extended leg back toward you (see Figure 10-5).**

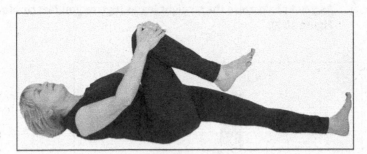

FIGURE 10-5:
Knee to chest.

3. **Stay for six to eight breaths and then switch and do the same with the left knee.**

Bent leg arm raise:

1. **Lie on your back with one leg bent and one leg straight, with your arms at your side.**

2. **As you inhale, bring both arms over your head (see Figure 10-6).**

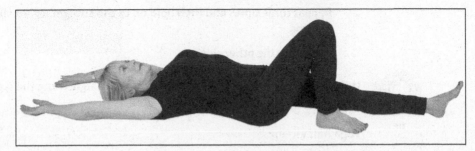

FIGURE 10-6:
Bent leg arm raise.

3. As you exhale, bring your arms back to your sides.

4. Repeat six to eight times slowly.

5. Repeat on the other side.

Straight leg hamstring stretch:

1. Lie on your back with your arms at your sides, palms down, and one leg bent with the foot on the ground.

2. Straighten the other leg.

3. As you exhale, raise the straight leg as high as you feel comfortable (see Figure 10-7).

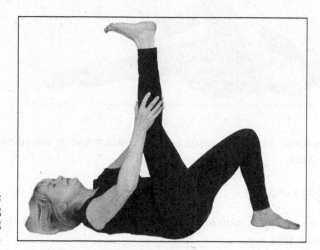

FIGURE 10-7: Straight leg hamstring stretch.

4. As you inhale, bring it back down.

5. Repeat three times and then hold on to the straight leg for six to eight breaths.

6. Repeat on the other side.

TIP

If this feels too challenging, try bending and straightening the leg you're holding on to (see Figure 10-8):

Yoga half sit-up:

1. Lie on your back with knees bent and feet on the ground.

2. Position a block, pillow, or folded blanket between your thighs, just below your knees.

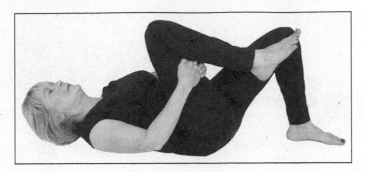

FIGURE 10-8:
Bent leg
hamstring
stretch.

3. **Place your thumbs at the top of your jaw and spread your fingers.**

4. **Take a deep breath and, as you exhale, squeeze your knees and sit just halfway up (see Figure 10-9).**

   TIP

   Don't throw the head forward; keep your arms wide. Let your eyes follow the ceiling.

5. **Inhale back and repeat six to eight times, gradually increasing repetitions to tolerance.**

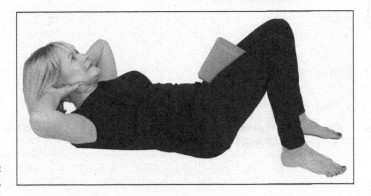

FIGURE 10-9:
Yoga half sit-up.

Yoga plank:

1. **Come to your hands and knees.**

2. **Slowly drop to your forearms and straighten your legs with your toes under (or the tops of your feet down) — see Figure 10-10.**

3. **Hold for six to eight breaths.**

TIP

You can gradually increase the hold time. Also, if this is too challenging starting out, try the same thing, but rest your knees on the ground (see Figure 10-11).

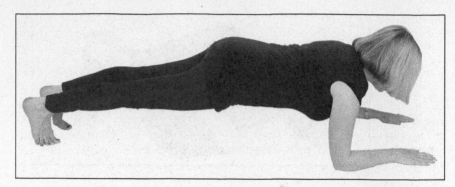

FIGURE 10-10:
Yoga plank.

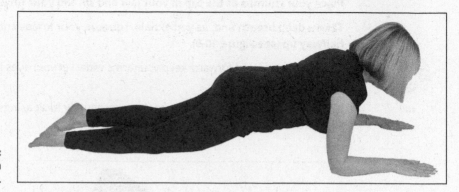

FIGURE 10-11:
Modified Yoga
plank.

Balancing cat:

1. **Start on your hands and knees.**

2. **Slide your left arm out and your right leg back, and then lift to be parallel with the floor (see Figure 10-12).**

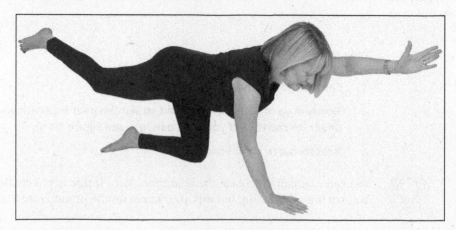

FIGURE 10-12:
Balancing cat.

3. **Stay for six to eight breaths.**

4. **Repeat on the other side.**

Lunge pose:

1. **Bring your right leg forward so that the right knee and ankle are in alignment; keep the left knee and foot on the ground.**

2. **Place your hands just above your right knee and straighten your back.**

3. **As you exhale lunge forward keeping your back straight (see Figure 10-13).**

4. **Repeat three times and then stay for six to eight breaths.**

   For greater intensity, tuck the tail under.

5. **Repeat on the other side.**

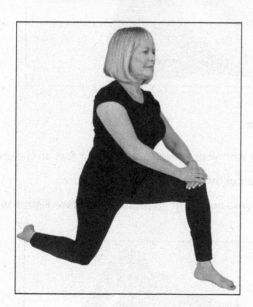

FIGURE 10-13: Lunge pose.

Knees to chest:

1. **Lie on your back and slowly bring your knees in toward your chest to tolerance (see Figure 10-14).**

   If you have knee problems, you can hold onto your legs underneath your thighs.

2. **Stay for six to eight breaths.**

TIP

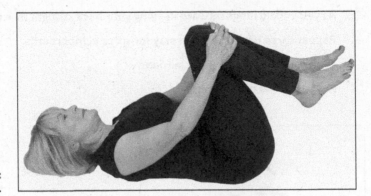

FIGURE 10-14:
Knees to chest.

Bent leg supine twist:

1. **Lie on you back with your knees bent and your feet on the ground.**

2. **Bring your arms out into a T with your palms down.**

3. **As you exhale, drop both bent knees to the left (see Figure 10-15).**

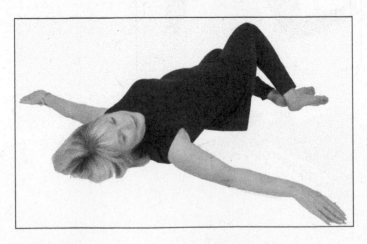

FIGURE 10-15:
Bent leg supine
twist.

4. **As you inhale, bring both knees up.**

5. **Repeat three times; on the third time, stay down for six to eight breaths.**

6. **Repeat on the other side.**

Knee to chest:

For the remainder of this routine, lie on your mat with your back to the floor.

1. **Lie on your back with both legs straight.**

2. **As you exhale, draw your right knee into your chest and bring the toes of your extended leg back toward you (see Figure 10-16).**

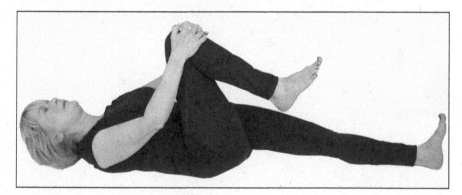

3. **Stay for six to eight breaths.**

4. **Do the same with the left leg.**

Attunement:

1. **Lie on your back with your knees bent, feet on the ground, and palms up (see Figure 10-17).**

2. **Breathe in and out through the nose 12 to 14 times.**

3. **Focus on linking your body, breath, and mind, which will help you to concentrate on what you're doing right now and keep your thoughts from wandering to other aspects of your life.**

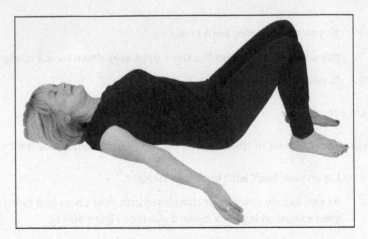

FIGURE 10-17:
Attunement.

IN THIS CHAPTER

» **Loosening tense muscles**

» **Improving your posture**

» **Combatting tension headaches**

» **Dealing with chronic asthma**

» **Doing Yoga that helps your upper back**

» **Trying Yogic breathing exercises**

Chapter **11**

Tending to Headaches, Asthma, and Your Upper Back

I n this chapter, I focus on your upper back and neck. So many ordinary lifestyle activities create problems in this area of the body, and Yoga can address some of those activities.

Tension headaches and chronic asthma may also respond favorably to the same Yoga routines that help your upper back. What all these conditions have in common is the need to

» Increase range of motion in your upper back and neck

» Open your chest

» Improve the way you are breathing

» Reduce stress

Yoga can help to loosen up chronically tense muscles in your upper back, neck, and shoulders. Maybe, more importantly, it helps to alleviate tension and stress, which is a common cause of many health problems.

WARNING

If you are in acute pain, you should first seek a diagnosis and relief in a doctor's office, not on a Yoga mat.

Age of Rounding

In Chapter 4, I first said that sitting is the new smoking — meaning that the act of doing too much sitting is affecting our health in a way that too much smoking once did.

And everybody sits.

Sitting too much can cause the spine to round. It's important to think about how often in your daily routines you round your back and how much sitting and other activities impact your body and posture (see Figure 11-1).

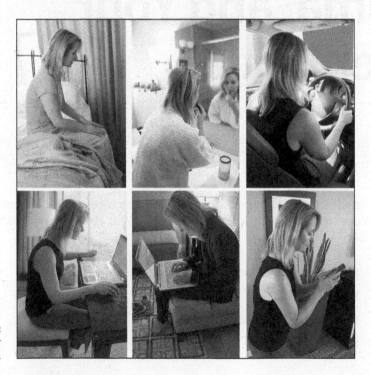

FIGURE 11-1:
Rounding your
back.

Consider the following points:

>> You sit on the edge of the bed when you first wake up.

>> You bend forward at the sink when getting ready for the day.

>> You drive to and from work (or someplace).

>> You sit at a desk or computer.

>> You spend more time rounding in front of your computer.

>> You round as you spend probably too much time on your phone.

Throughout all of these activities, you round your back and the muscles in your chest (your pectorals) get shorter. As a result, over time, you start to round forward. Yoga helps reverse this rounding by stretching your chest muscles, giving you a straighter posture.

Tension and Stress

If there's one thing I probably don't need to sell you on, it's that tension and stress are prevalent forces. If you consider the most common causes of stress, it's pretty clear that no one is immune:

>> Relationship problems, divorce, or lack of a desired relationship

>> Job-related stress or job loss

>> Money issues

>> A home or office move

>> Serious illness or injury

>> Caregiving of a family member

>> Death of a loved one

>> Being a victim of crime

Among my student population, I can think of at least one person who fits into each of these categories. But if tension and stress are common human experiences, what is not common is how to deal with it all successfully. Some lucky people seem to let stress roll off of them like a gentle rain. Other people become completely overwhelmed. Once again, Yoga offers a way to transcend emotional suffering by calming the nervous system and releasing feel-good hormones.

Tension Headaches

While any number of things can trigger a headache, certainly tension and stress are common culprits.

Tension headaches often feel like a tight pressure that surrounds the head and squeezes. These types of headaches are usually felt on both sides of the head at the same time and are a steady ache.

The pain associated with a tension headache can be anywhere from mild to excruciating. These kinds of headaches can be debilitating.

Oftentimes, headaches develop near the end of a stressful day. Of course, if you carry your stress with you throughout the night you may wake up with a tension headache. The bottom line is that stress is like jet fuel to these types of headaches.

Because practicing Yoga is a way to reduce stress, it can also be used as a powerful tool to fight the tension associated with tension headaches.

Breathing for Better Health

This chapter focuses on stretching and loosening the muscles in the neck, back, and shoulders, which are some of the same muscles used in the ordinary act of breathing. Simply stated, loosening the muscles in this part of the body will help you to breathe. And if you're dealing with the symptoms of asthma or Chronic Obstructive Pulmonary Disease (COPD), these practices may help.

You've been breathing on your own for a long time, and you probably think you don't need me to give you lessons. Still, you may have developed breathing patterns that aren't as efficient as they could be. And this issue may especially ring true for people suffering from COPD, asthma, or other obstructive disorders, such as chronic bronchitis or emphysema.

Yoga breathing exercises sometimes focus on using the diaphragm more in the process of breathing. By engaging the diaphragm, you may be able to exhale more completely — a goal, to be sure, for people who suffer from asthma or COPD.

Diaphragmatic breathing

I have avoided, for the most part, discussions of anatomy in this book. However, keep in mind that with every breath you take, your lungs fill up with air and your diaphragm descends into your abdominal cavity. By developing breathing habits that minimize the diaphragm's involvement in the respiratory process, you're severely limiting the power of your own breath.

Breathing with full movement of the diaphragm can actually increase the relaxation response, which in turn reduces the stress and tension that can build up in the neck, shoulders, and back — those areas of the body that are the focus of this chapter. Moreover, for COPD and asthma sufferers, diminished lung capacity and breathing function can cause these areas of the upper back to tighten up in response.

Belly breathing routine

The home routine in the following sections can help your upper back (or to keep it healthy). First, though, give this simple belly breathing a try.

1. **Lie flat on your back and place one hand on your chest and the other on your abdomen.**

    Your hand position helps you detect motion during belly breathing.

2. **Place a small pillow or folded blanket under your head if you have tension in your neck or if your chin tilts upward.**

3. **Place a large pillow under your knees if your back is uncomfortable.**

4. **During inhalation, expand your abdomen; during exhalation, contract your abdomen but keep your chest as motionless as possible.**

    Again, your hands act as motion detectors.

5. **Pause for a couple of seconds between inhalation and exhalation, keeping the throat soft.**

6. **Take 15 to 20 slow, deep breaths.**

At-Home Routine for Upper Back

The following routine basically contains the same sequence that I recently provided to students and staff at a major medical school. The poses in this sequence are especially good for helping maintain a healthy back.

WARNING

Please consult with your doctor before beginning — especially if you're experiencing acute pain.

Focus breathing:

1. **Sit comfortably in an armless chair with your back nice and tall; place your palms comfortably on your thighs.**

2. **Look straight ahead and bring your head comfortably back until the middle of your ears, your shoulders, and your hip sockets are in alignment, as shown in Figure 11-2.**

3. **With your eyes open or closed, stay for six to eight breaths.**

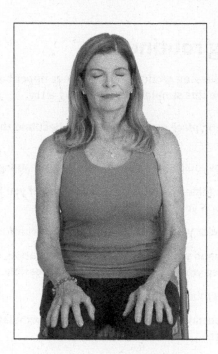

FIGURE 11-2:
Focus breathing.

Seated alternate arm raise:

1. **Start in the seated chair posture.**

2. **As you inhale, raise your right arm, as shown in Figure 11-3.**

3. **As you exhale, return your right palm to your right thigh; repeat Steps 2 and 3, alternating with your right and left arms two to three times each.**

Seated alternate arm raise with head turn:

1. **Continue the previous movements, with the following variation.**

2. **As you inhale, raise your right arm and turn your head to the left (see Figure 11-4).**

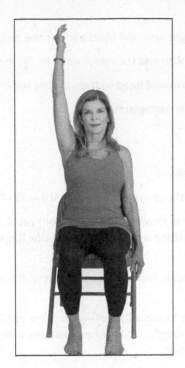

FIGURE 11-3:
Seated alternate arm raise.

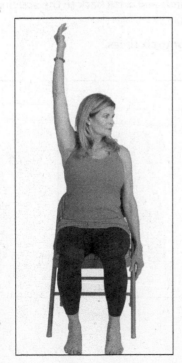

FIGURE 11-4:
Seated alternate arm raise with head turn.

3. As you exhale, bring your right arm and head back to the center.

4. As you inhale, raise the left arm and turn your head to the right.

5. Exhale as you return your arm and head to the starting position.

6. Repeat four to six times, alternating arms.

Wing and a prayer (extended):

1. Start in the seated chair posture.

2. Join your palms together in the prayer position, as shown in Figure 11-5a.

3. As you inhale, raise your arms comfortably above your head, keeping your hands in the prayer position and your eyes on your fingertips (see Figure 11-5b).

4. As you exhale, bring your hands and arms back down, still maintaining the prayer position.

5. As you inhale, separate your hands and move your arms out like wings to the sides at about shoulder height, lifting your chest and looking straight ahead, as shown in Figure 11-5c.

6. As you exhale, bring your hands and arms back to the starting position (prayer hands at your chest).

7. Repeat Steps 1 through 6 four to six times.

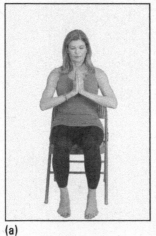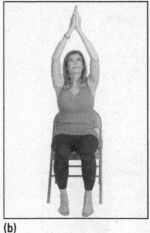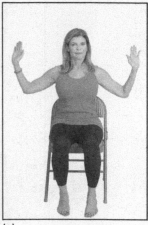

FIGURE 11-5: Wing and prayer (extended).

(a)　　　　　　　　　(b)　　　　　　　　　(c)

Mirror on hand:

1. **Start in the seated chair posture.**

2. **As you inhale, raise the back of your right hand to eye level, as shown in Figure 11-6a.**

3. **As you exhale, bring your right hand inward and place your palm and fingers at the top of your left shoulder, turning your eyes and head down and to the left as you follow your right hand (see Figure 11-6b).**

WARNING

If you have a problem rotating your neck outward to the right or the left, only turn as far as you feel comfortable.

4. **As you inhale, return the back of your right hand to eye level and keep it moving and opening around to the right as far as is comfortable (see Figure 11-6c).**

5. **As you exhale, bring the back of the right hand in front of you again at eye level (like you did in Figure 11-6a).**

6. **Continue exhaling as you bring the right hand back down to the seated chair posture (see Figure 11-6d).**

7. **Repeat Steps 1 through 6, alternating right and left sides three to four times each.**

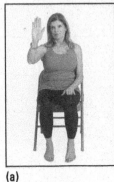 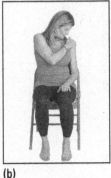 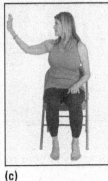 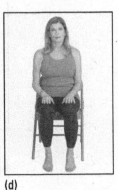

FIGURE 11-6:
Mirror on hand. (a)　　　　　(b)　　　　　(c)　　　　　(d)

Shoulder rolls:

1. Start in the seated chair posture.

2. Hang your arms at your sides and roll your shoulders up and back as you inhale (see Figure 11-7).

3. As you exhale, roll your shoulders down.

4. Repeat Steps 2 and 3 four to six times and then reverse the direction of the rolls for four to six repetitions.

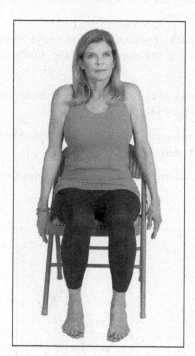

Bent arm shoulder rolls:

1. Extend your arms out in front of you with your palms up.

2. Bend your elbows and bring your fingertips to your shoulders. (see Figure 11-8a)

3. With your elbows, make big circles in one direction (see Figure 11-8b).

4. After making 5 rotations, reverse the direction of your circles.

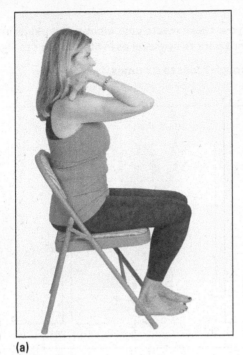
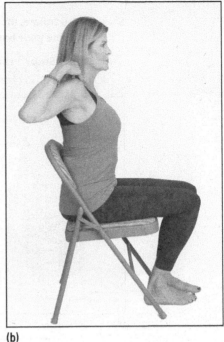

FIGURE 11-8:
Bent arm
shoulder rolls.   (a)   (b)

Newspaper:

1. **Start in the seated chair posture.**

2. **Inhale and then, as you exhale, move both hands up to eye level with your palms facing you as though you were looking at a newspaper (see Figure 11-9a).**

3. **As you inhale, move both hands up and follow your hands with your eyes and head until your hands are just above your forehead, as shown in Figure 11-9b.**

TIP

Try not to turn your head too far back when you're looking up at your hands. Think of rotating up from the level of your ears rather than your collar.

4. **As you exhale, bring your chin down to your chest without moving your arms, as shown in Figure 11-9c.**

5. **As you inhale, separate your hands and move your arms out like wings to the sides at about shoulder height, lifting your chest and looking straight ahead (see Figure 11-9d).**

6. **As you exhale, extend your bent arms forward like they're going over a log and round your back like a camel as you look down (see Figure 11-9e).**

7. As you inhale, lift your chest; rotate your elbows and palms inward as you raise your hands back to eye level as in Step 2 (refer to Figure 11-9a).

8. Repeat Steps 1 through 7 four to six times.

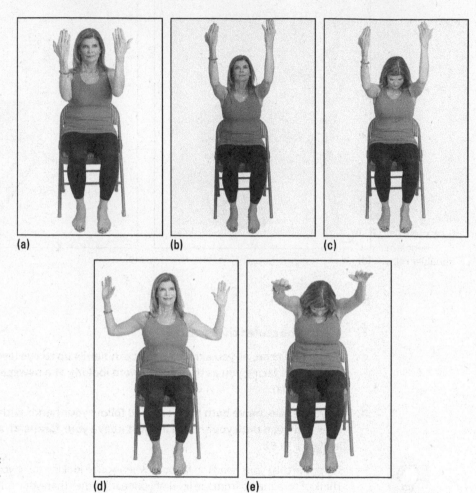

FIGURE 11-9:
Newspaper.

Seated chair twist:

 WARNING

In the following seated chair twist, resist the temptation to crank this twist too hard. Move slowly and carefully. If you experience pain or discomfort, leave the twist out of your routine and check with your health professional.

1. Start in the seated chair posture turned sideways with the back of the chair to your right; hold the sides of the chair back with your hands (see Figure 11-10).

2. As you inhale, extend or lift your spine and head upward.

3. As you exhale, twist your torso and head farther to the right.

4. Repeat Steps 2 and 3, gradually twisting to your comfort level, and then stay in the twist for four to six breaths.

5. Repeat Steps 1 through 4 on the left side.

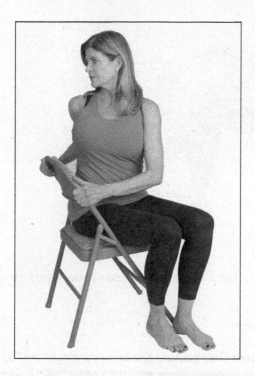

FIGURE 11-10:
Seated chair
twist.

Seated fold:

1. Start in the seated chair posture turned sideways with the chair back on either your left or right.

2. As you exhale, bend forward from the hips and slide your hands down your legs as you hang your head, chest, and arms comfortably, as shown in Figure 11-11.

WARNING

Keep your back straight if rounding causes you pain (regardless of how far forward you come).

3. Stay in Step 2 for six to eight breaths.

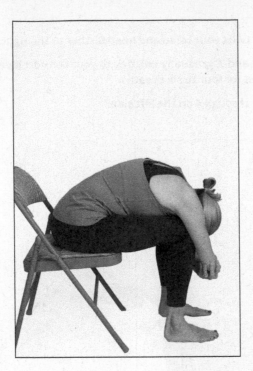

FIGURE 11-11:
Seated fold.

WARNING

If it's too painful to bend forward, you may choose to arch your back as an alternative.

Shoulder self-massage:

1. Start in the seated chair posture and bring your right arm up and across toward your left shoulder; place your right palm down between the top of your left shoulder and your neck, as shown in Figure 11-12.

2. Slowly and gently massage the surface area between the neck and the left shoulder in a circular motion (starting toward the neck) six to eight times, noticing any tight spots.

3. Find the tightest spot you identified in Step 2 and grab or squeeze each one firmly for six to eight counts.

4. Finish the self-massage by repeating Step 2 six to eight times.

5. Repeat Steps 1 through 4 with the left hand on your right side.

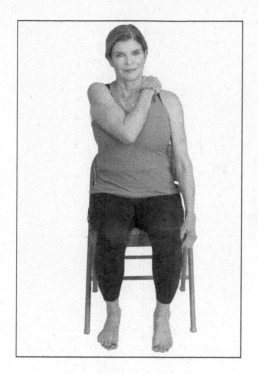

Seated belly breathing:

1. Start in the seated chair posture with your either opened eyes closed (see Figure 11-13).

2. Use belly breathing and gradually increase the length of your exhalation until you reach your comfortable maximum.

   See more on belly breathing in the preceding section.

3. Take 20 to 30 belly breaths and then gradually come back to your normal breath.

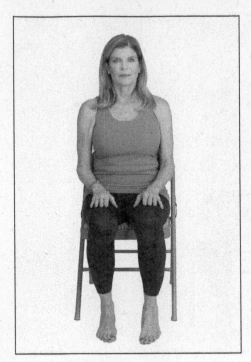

FIGURE 11-13:
Seated belly
breathing.

Chapter **12**

Dealing with Needy Knees

This chapter focuses on your knees. Knee problems usually become more prevalent with age. That's not surprising because we ask a lot from these joints. They absorb significant pressure created by your own body weight, particularly in the act of taking simple steps down the stairway or sidewalk. Unfortunately, over time, the knees themselves can start to deteriorate.

The goal is to slow down the deterioration of your knees, the weakening of muscles and ligaments, and the disintegration of cartilage. Yoga offers some interventions that may help prevent or at least delay this process. You can find out more about joint replacements in Chapter 14 and arthritis in Chapter 16.

Are Your Knees Making a Crackling Noise?

When I'm teaching a Yoga class and the student demographic tends to fall into the 50-and-above range, it never fails to happen: I'll ask people to come into some kind of squat, and the room suddenly reverberates with the sound of creaking bones — it's what I like to call the sound of "maturing knees."

In some cases, the crackling noise you hear coming from your joints — especially your knees — is called *crepitus*. Crepitus basically describes a condition where, due to normal wear, the tendons or ligaments actually snap over the bony structures of the knee or the joint surface.

Crepitus is the grinding, cracking, or crunching sound you hear when bending your knees. And, yes, it is yet another reward for getting older; crepitus definitely becomes more common as we age.

REMEMBER

Crepitus is part of the natural aging process of the joints and, unless accompanied by pain or swelling, is probably harmless.

If you're noticing other symptoms — especially pain — you should consult your healthcare provider. Something more serious, such as arthritis, may be going on with your knee joints.

Yoga can help your knees stay healthy

Yoga offers a multitude of health benefits for your knees.

The knee itself is a relatively simple joint (a hinge joint, in this case) and even without injury, arthritis, or other conditions, normal wear and tear will take its toll. You can, however, use a regular Yoga practice to help build the surrounding muscles that support the knee joints. These muscles include:

>> Quadriceps

>> Hamstrings

>> Hip abductor and hip external rotator muscles, plus hip flexor and adductor muscles

>> Feet and ankle muscles

Like any joints, the knees are challenged by weight-bearing postures. Using your body weight helps build the muscles around the knees, but body weight can put a load on the joints — another reason I make a pitch for keeping your weight down.

Sadly, I often need to correct my Yoga students because they go into postures without considering the proper alignment of their knees. Making the same mistakes, week after week, will eventually do damage. Finding and maintaining proper knee alignment when practicing Yoga is essential.

Because the knees are hinge joints, they are designed to move back and forth (to flex and straighten) and not move from side to side. There's not much in the knee itself to stop that side movement from happening, so the knees depend on the surrounding muscles and ligaments to keep them in place. But as any football player knows, that doesn't always happen, and injury can keep you off the field — or off your Yoga mat.

The most important thing you can do to protect your knees is to make sure they're tracking right over your feet when they bend. Your knees should move in the same direction that your toes are pointing (see Figure 12-1).

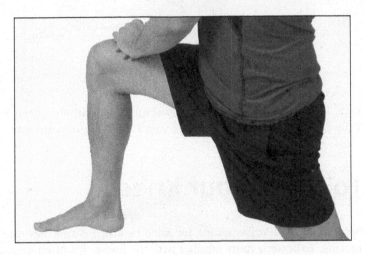

FIGURE 12-1:
Knees track over toes.

You can also keep a slight bend in your knees at all times if you tend to lock-out the joint or hyperextend. While the knees allow you to straighten your legs, some hypermobile people are more prone to hyperextension, which can lead to joint damage.

Smarter, not tougher

Always feel free to cushion your knees whenever you need to be on all fours (hands and knees) or to stand on your knees (see Figure 12-2). This advice is particularly helpful if you happen to be practicing on a wooden or tile floor. That quarter-inch thick (or less) Yoga mat is definitely not enough of a cushion. Adding a folded blanket, for example, underneath your kneecaps may make a lot of sense.

Some people believe using a blanket under their knees is somehow cheating, but that couldn't be further from the truth. Using a cushion may allow you to get into the pose more quickly and stay in it longer.

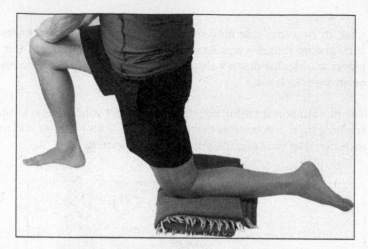

FIGURE 12-2:
Cushioning your
knees.

REMEMBER

Your knees are actually very bony structures, without much built-in padding.
Take care of them now so that you won't develop problems later.

Getting to Know Your Knees

Before you do a Yoga routine for knee health, I'd first like you to do this pre-routine. To become more familiar with the knees, it's often informative to understand your knee anatomy.

TIP

1. **Sit comfortably on the floor or put a blanket or bolster underneath your hips you so that you can sit comfortably.**

   Extend your legs out in front of you.

2. **Place your hands on your thighs, with one hand on each leg, and just rub up and down a few times over those big muscles called the quadriceps.**

3. **Put your hands underneath your thighs and feel the muscles that go from the back of your knee up to the buttocks.**

   These muscles are your hamstrings.

4. **Bring your hands to the muscles on the insides of your upper legs, which are your adductors.**

5. **Move your hands to the outside of your upper legs, feeling up and down.**

   These muscles are called your abductors.

6. **Bring your hands upward to your hips and then your buttocks.**

7. **Place your hands below your knees and feel the calf muscles (behind your shins).**

8. **Put your hands directly on your knees (see Figure 12-3).**

   Notice how small they feel and just how much they are controlled by the other surrounding muscles. When it comes to knee usage, it is certainly a team effort!

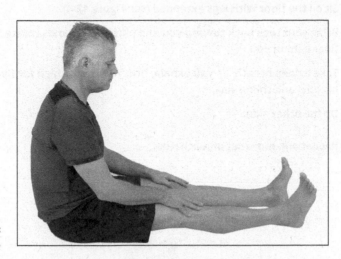

FIGURE 12-3:
Feel your knees.

Yoga Routine for Your Knees

I talk a lot about breathing in Chapter 3. It's the breath, after all, that makes Yoga such a unique discipline in the first place.

So, as you prepare to do the following knee sequence, start off by doing some simple focus breathing as described in the following steps (in any comfortable position). See Chapter 3 for a larger discussion on focus breathing.

REMEMBER

During your Yoga practice, simply follow the directions I give you about when to inhale and exhale.

1. **Breathe only through the nose and make the breath a little longer than normal.**

   That's all you have to do! Don't worry about where the breath is starting or ending; just breathe slowly and evenly.

2. After you're used to this type of breathing, add a short pause of one or two seconds after the inhalation and another one after exhalation.

3. When you feel ready, add drawing the belly in during exhalation without force or exaggeration.

Yoga quad sets:

1. Sit on the floor with legs extended (see Figure 12-4).

2. Bring your toes back toward you and place both hands rotated out on the floor behind you.

3. Take a deep breath; as you exhale, firm your right thigh for five to seven breaths and then relax.

4. Do the other side.

5. Repeat one more set on each side.

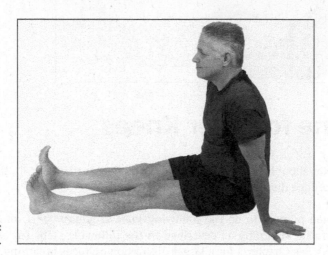

FIGURE 12-4:
Yoga quad sets.

Boat pose variation:

1. Sit on the floor with legs extended, toes back, and both hands rotated out on the floor behind you.

2. As you exhale, firm the right thigh and lift it to the height of your toes on your left foot (see Figure 12-5).

3. Point and flex the right foot; stay for five to seven breaths.

    You can lean back a little if it's more comfortable.

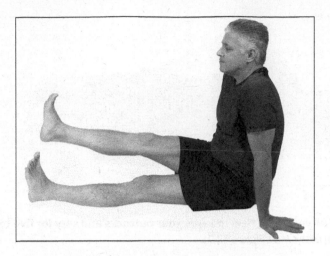

FIGURE 12-5:
Boat pose
variation.

4. **Repeat on the other side.**

5. **Repeat one more set on each side.**

Side reclining bow variation:

1. **Lie on your left side with your left hand under your head or a pillow or blanket (see Figure 12-6).**

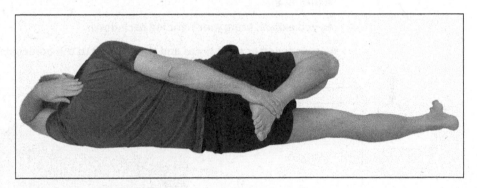

FIGURE 12-6:
Side reclining
bow variation.

2. **Straighten both legs.**

3. **Bend your right (top) leg at the knee.**

4. **Reach back with your right hand and hold the right foot or ankle.**

   If you can't reach your foot, use a strap or towel (see Figure 12-7).

TIP

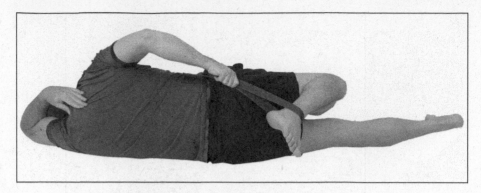

FIGURE 12-7:
Using a strap.

5. **Pull your right heel towards your buttocks and stay for five to seven breaths (see Figure 12-7).**

To avoid pain or injury, be careful not to twist your thigh or leg outward.

WARNING

6. **Repeat on the other side.**

Side reclining leg lift variation:

1. **Lie on your left side with your left hand under your head (or use a pillow or folded blanket).**

2. **As you inhale, raise right leg to your comfortable maximum (see Figure 12-8).**

3. **As you exhale, bring your right leg back down.**

4. **Repeat seven or eight times and then switch to the other side.**

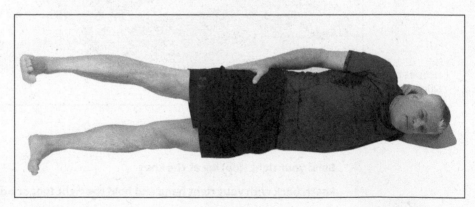

FIGURE 12-8:
Side reclining leg
lift variation.

Bridge pose modification:

1. Lie on your back with your knees bent and your hands at your sides, palms down.

2. Place a block or folded pillow horizontally between your groin and knees (see Figure 12-9).

3. As you inhale, squeeze the block and raise your hips to your comfort level.

4. As you exhale, lower your hips back down.

5. Repeat three times and then stay up for six to eight breaths.

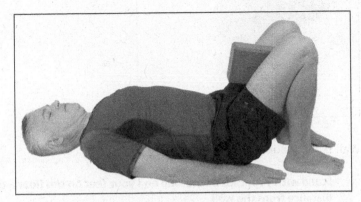

FIGURE 12-9:
Bridge pose
modification.

Chair pose with the wall:

1. Stand with your back, hips, and head (if possible) to a wall and your feet a comfortable distance away (preparing for a half squat).

2. As you inhale, raise your hands and arms parallel to the floor.

3. As you exhale, slide halfway down keeping your back and head at the wall.

   Make sure your knees are in a 90-degree angle with your ankles (see Figure 12-10).

REMEMBER

4. Repeat three times and then stay for six to eight breaths.

5. (Optional) Do a second set if you are up to it.

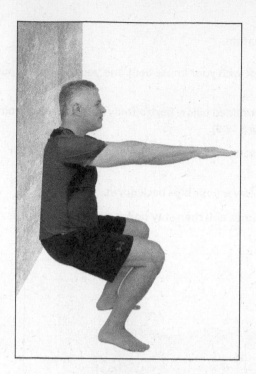

FIGURE 12-10:
Chair pose
modification.

Wall hang (modified forward bend):

1. **Stand with your hips at the wall and your feet on the floor a comfortable distance from the wall.**

2. **As you exhale, simply hang down and hold your elbows with opposite hands (see Figure 12-11).**

3. **Let the wall support your hips so that you can soften your knees, release your back, neck, and head, and really relax.**

4. **Stay for 8 to 12 breaths.**

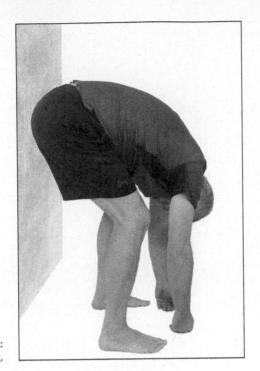

FIGURE 12-11:
Wall hang.

Chapter 13

Handling Hopeful Hips and Hamstrings

About ten years ago, the Mayo Clinic published a study that warned of the health dangers associated with too much sitting. Almost a decade later, people are still sitting more than ever — and the impact on postures and backs grows more and more ominous as hips and hamstrings continue to get tighter.

The effect of all this sitting gets even more menacing as you age. Tight or stiffening hamstring and hip muscles may not only be the cause of routine pain; they can also be at the root of various back issues.

Of course, these muscles are part of the whole chain that helps you move from place to place. So, keep in mind that problems with your hips and hamstrings may also show up in your lower body, including your knees and feet.

It's All in the Hips

I don't want to turn this book into an anatomy class, but here's a fun fact: Your hips are one of the biggest structures in your body. When I talk about *hips*, I'm talking about the

>> Pelvis

>> Lower back (sacrum)

>> Upper legs (femurs)

>> Muscles and ligaments that hold them all together while allowing them to move

The hips also include those two large sockets that hold the tops of your legs (your *femurs*) in place. (These ball-and-socket joints are considered by some to be the largest joints in your body.)

REMEMBER

Your hips allow your legs to swing back and forth as you walk or run. But because your hips are made up of ball joints, your legs can actually move in all directions. A multitude of muscles and ligaments support this wide range of motion and, at the same time, keep your legs safely attached.

All these surrounding muscles can become tight and even painful to move. That's where Yoga comes in.

REMEMBER

Other chapters in this book talk about the degeneration of certain joints, and certainly the hips are often the targets of joint replacements. In this chapter, however, I just want to talk to you about keeping your hips healthy.

Bearing the Weight

You can easily see that the structure of your hips is actually quite complex and, by comparison to other bodily structures, quite massive, as well. Your hips are designed to support your entire upper body weight as you walk, run, dance, or play basketball — and the hip joints, themselves are one of the largest weight-bearing joints in your body.

Supporting these joints are a series of muscles that need to remain flexible and strong, including:

>> Gluteals

>> Adductors and abductors

>> Iliopsoas

>> Quadriceps (the front of your thigh)

Without overwhelming you with anatomical terminology, I want to make the point that when I'm talking about the hips, I'm talking about a lot of different parts that need to stay toned and mobile.

In that regard, let me add to the list the *iliotibial band* (or IT band). The IT band is a long tendon attached to several hip and thigh muscles. Sometimes, this tendon can become too tight or overused, and it can cause hip problems.

Any of these muscles can be *tight* — immobile or inflexible due to things like inactivity or too much sitting (in the car, on the couch in front of the TV, or at your desk in front of your computer). And, in addition to sitting, other relatively innocuous activities can lead to some pretty serious hip pain.

Hamstrings

Hamstrings are located on the back of your thighs and consist of three different muscles that support both the hip joints and the knee joints.

If you're going to keep your hamstrings flexible and strong, be aware that each one is made up of three distinct muscles. Oftentimes, postures that are intended to target hamstring muscles focus mostly on the muscle that runs up the center of the back leg, putting less emphasis on the inner and outer hamstring muscles. (I avoid that mistake in the home routine that appears at the end of this chapter.)

Because the hamstrings support both the hip and knee joints, you'll want to keep your hamstrings strong and flexible in the first place. If hips and knees help you walk and run, the support that the hamstrings give both of these structures is invaluable.

Yoga teachers and Yoga therapists I've talked with agree that the hamstrings are one muscle group that prevents many people from folding forward beyond their knees or straightening legs to the ceiling when lying on their back. Of course, how far one goes in any pose is irrelevant, but human nature is such that people want to achieve a position's full range.

So tight hamstrings can be very restrictive — particularly inhibiting the hips from hinging forward. Unfortunately, many people try to compensate for their hips' inability to allow for a deep forward fold by using their spines. This can cause back strain or worse, even injuries.

Be thoughtful when you bend forward and understand that when your hips stop tilting, you need to stop trying.

A Hips and Hamstrings Sequence for Home

Before you begin this home routine, start with some belly breathing (see Chapter 3) and keep this pattern of breathing throughout the following routine:

1. **Lie flat on your back and place one hand on your chest and the other on your abdomen.**

   Place a small pillow or folded blanket under your head if you have tension in your neck or if your chin tilts upward. Place a large pillow under your knees if your back is uncomfortable. Your hand position helps you detect motion during belly breathing.

2. **Inhale, expanding your abdomen; exhale, contracting your abdomen.**

3. **Pause for a couple of seconds between inhalation and exhalation, keeping the throat soft.**

4. **Take 10 to 15 slow, deep breaths.**

Bound angle pose at the wall:

1. **Sit on the floor with your back to a wall.**

   Use blankets or pillows under your hips if you need them.

2. **Bend your knees and join your feet together; let your knees drop down to their comfort level (see Figure 13-1).**

3. **Stay for six to eight breaths.**

Legs up the wall series:

1. **Lie on your back with both legs up the wall and your hips at a comfortable distance from the wall; let your arms rest comfortably at your sides with palms down.**

2. **As you inhale, let just the right leg down slowly toward the floor (see Figure 13-2a).**

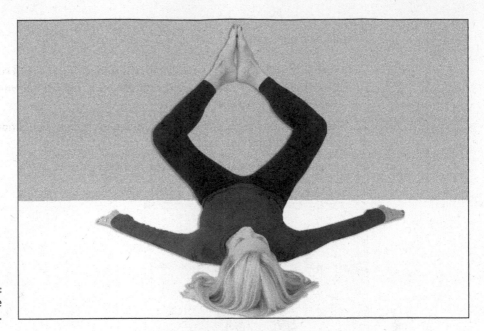

FIGURE 13-1:
Bound angle pose
at the wall.

3. As you exhale, slowly bring it back up.

4. Repeat on the left side.

5. Open both legs at the wall and until you reach a comfortable distance from the floor (see Figure 13-2b).

6. Stay for 6 to 8 breaths and slowly work up to 12 to 16 breaths.

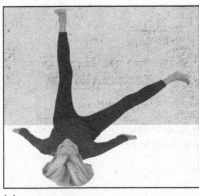
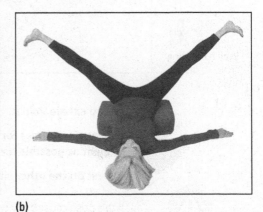

FIGURE 13-2:
Legs up the wall.
(a)

(b)

Wall hamstring series:

1. Stay on your back near the wall and, without giving yourself rug burn, move back enough that you can have your feet flat on the wall with your shins parallel with the floor.

2. Keep your left foot at the wall and use both hands to hold underneath your right thigh.

3. As you inhale, straighten your right leg (see Figure 13-3).

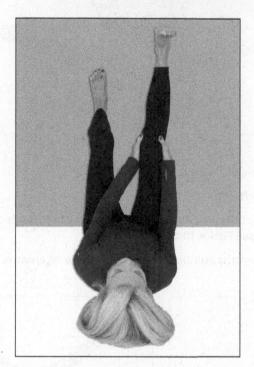

FIGURE 13-3:
Wall hamstring series.

4. As you exhale, fold it.

5. Repeat three times for a total of four; on the last one, hold your leg as straight as possible for six to eight breaths.

6. Repeat on the other side.

WARNING

If this pose causes any type of pain, skip the pose altogether.

Windshield wiper:

1. **Start on your back away from the wall with your knees bent and feet wide on the ground.**

2. **Bring your arms into a T not higher than your shoulders, with your palms facing down.**

3. **As you exhale, drop both knees to the right. (See Figure 13-4.)**

   To protect your hip joint, do not do this pose if it causes you pinching or pain.

WARNING

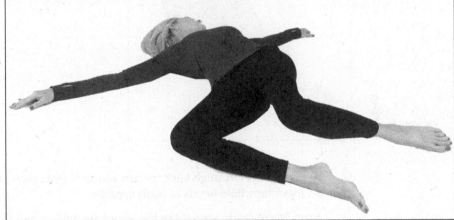

FIGURE 13-4: Windshield wiper.

4. **As you inhale, bring both knees up.**

5. **As you exhale, drop both knees to the left.**

6. **Repeat three times for a total of four on each side and then stay down on one side for six to eight breaths.**

7. **Flip your knees to the other side and hold again for six to eight breaths.**

   To make it more challenging, place the side of the ankle of the inside foot on top of the opposite knee for a deeper stretch.

TIP

Reclined cow face variation sequence:

1. **Lie on your back with your knees bent and feet comfortably apart on the ground.**

2. **Place the outside of your right ankle just above the left knee.**

3. **Slide your right hand through the opening and use both hands to hold the back of your left thigh (see Figure 13-5).**

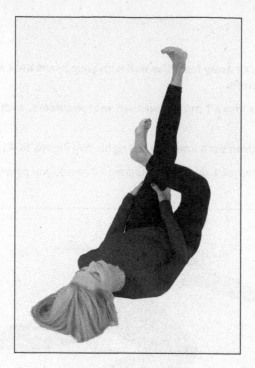

FIGURE 13-5:
Reclined figure four variation.

4. Slowly pull the left thigh back toward you until you reach your comfortable maximum; hold for six to eight breaths.

5. When you're ready, straighten the leg you're holding and then bend it again for three to five times.

6. Repeat on the other side.

WARNING

If this pose causes any type of pain, reduce the intensity of the stretch or skip the pose altogether.

Happy baby sequence:

1. Lie on your back with your arms comfortably at your sides, palms down, and your knees bent with your feet on the floor.

2. Join the soles of your feet together and let your bent knees drop toward the floor (to your comfort level); stay for four to five breaths.

3. Bring your feet and bent knees toward your belly and reach up to hold your ankles or your feet with both hands; stay for four to five breaths (see Figure 13-6).

4. Continue to hold the outsides of both ankles or feet, but separate them and bring your knees toward the floor.

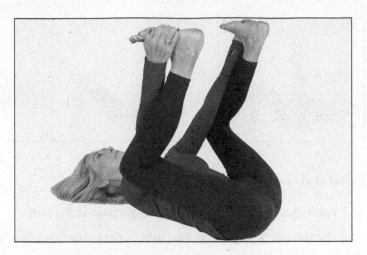

FIGURE 13-6:
Happy baby pose.

5. **Stay for four to five breaths and gently rock from side to side a few times.**

6. **Bring the soles of your feet back together and hold them for four to five breaths.**

7. **Bring the joined soles of your feet back to the ground for four to five breaths.**

This hamstring trifecta routine addresses all three hamstring muscles:

1. **Lie on your back with your left leg bent, foot on the ground, and your right leg straight (with your toes pointing back toward you).**

2. **As you exhale, bring your right leg up.**

3. **As you inhale, take it back down.**

4. **Repeat for a total of three times and then hold your right leg up for four to five breaths (or until you reach your comfortable maximum).**

   If you have difficulty holding your leg or foot, use a strap or towel.

TIP

5. **Move your right leg away from your midline (the imaginary line that runs through the center of your body top to bottom) about a foot then backwards from that position; stay for four to five breaths (see Figure 13-7).**

6. **Move your right leg across your midline to the inside.**

   Be careful as you now pull the leg backwards from this inside position.

   Back off if anything feels painful.

WARNING

7. **Repeat the entire process on the other side.**

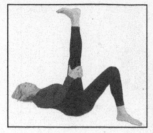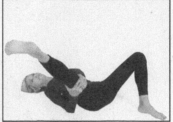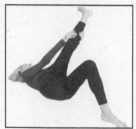

FIGURE 13-7:
Hamstring
trifecta.

Bound angle pose at the wall to finish:

1. **Finish this routine with the bound angle pose at the wall.**

   This is the same pose as the first pose you did in this series. (See Figure 13-8.)

2. **Continue to use belly breathing, now trying to make your exhales longer.**

   Notice if you have made some progress with how the hips open.

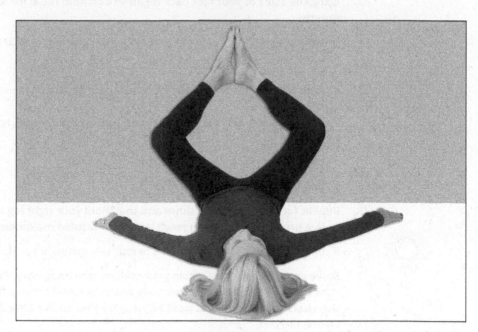

FIGURE 13-8:
Bound angle pose
at the wall.

Chapter **14**

Dealing with Joint Replacements

S ometimes a joint — often the hip or knee joint — wears out, and the only way to fix it is with a joint replacement. In this chapter, I discuss practicing Yoga after you have had this type of surgery.

I do want to make clear that this chapter deals specifically with joint replacements. If you want to read more about how Yoga can help to keep your hips and knees healthy, see Chapter 13.

And please, before doing any Yoga after a joint replacement, check with your healthcare provider. I am not a medical doctor and cannot prescribe your rehab.

Refining Your Yoga Practice

The surgical procedures and the materials used to build new joints are getting better all the time. As medical technology gallops forward, surgeons must refine their techniques, and it is equally important for you to refine how you practice Yoga.

Your objective is to provide as much support as possible to the new joint (perhaps by stretching or strengthening the surrounding muscles and ligaments) and not strain or stress the new joint by asking it to perform movements that may unduly stress it.

Your surgeon and physical therapist (PT) will provide you with a lot of advice on what postures or movements are safe to perform and what will be rehabilitative. If you want to include Yoga in your fitness regime — either starting a new practice or picking back up on an old one — you simply need to listen to your doctor, your PT, your Yoga teacher, and, of course, your own body.

You should do Yoga only when your healthcare providers tell you it's okay (usually 8 to 12 weeks after surgery, but that can vary).

Hip Replacements

The goal in any Yoga practice, especially if you've had a hip replacement, is to stay safe and minimize the risk of injury, including dislocating your new joint. The key to safe Yoga with a hip replacement is knowing the type of surgery you had: posterior or anterior. Just this fact will determine the types of postures and movements that are safe, as well as those you should avoid.

When a surgeon performs a hip replacement, the point of entry used to be exclusively from the back *(posterior)*. The incision is in the upper part of the thigh, either along the outside or along the back side, and it typically required cutting through muscles.

A newer procedure allows the surgeon to enter the hip area through the front of the thigh *(anterior)*. This approach cuts fewer muscles and ultimately allows for a faster recovery.

While it certainly does matter if your surgery was an anterior or posterior procedure, I recommend caution in both cases. You obviously want to avoid any movements that risk joint dislocation. In addition to the type of procedure you had, a big factor in joint vulnerability has to do with how long ago your surgery occurred.

To be on the safe side, avoid any pose that's going to take your range of motion to an extreme. And, when in doubt, ask your doctor.

If you're naturally very flexible (you may even be considered *double jointed* or *hypermobile*), you may be prone to joint dislocation. You should focus your Yoga practice on strength building and avoid the deeper or sustained stretches around your artificial joint, which was not designed to replicate your previous level of flexibility.

Anterior replacements

WARNING

If your hip replacement was done using the anterior method, where your surgeon enters your hip through the front, you will want to avoid the following movements:

>> Extension (bending backwards at the hip or taking a long step backwards, as in lunges)

>> External rotation (turning your thighs outward or crossing the ankle over the opposite knee)

>> Abduction (moving your leg outward — though this movement may be okay if it's not painful)

You should also probably avoid the following poses:

>> Child's pose (or any pose that requires the full weight of the body pushing the joint to the end of its range of motion)

>> Triangle (abduction and external rotation)

>> Warrior I (extension of one hip)

>> Warrior II (extension/abduction and external rotation)

>> Most standing backbends (extension of one or both hips)

>> Bound angle (external rotation and abduction)

>> Lotus (extreme external rotation)

After any form of hip surgery, you will probably work with a physical therapist during the acute stage, which can be 6 to 12 weeks or more, depending on your personal recovery time.

After the acute stage, with the anterior approach, you will normally have more range of motion than with the posterior approach (see the next section). Of course, the idea is to avoid what feels like extremes of motion or causes pain.

The tissues at the front of the hip can remain tight for several months following an anterior hip replacement, or the muscle that brings the knee toward the head (hip flexor) can be weak. This tightness or weakness usually resolves with time, and your physical therapist or rehab professional will guide you through rehabilitative exercises.

Posterior replacements

WARNING

If your hip replacement was done using the more traditional posterior procedure, which is from the back, you will want to avoid the following movements:

>> Internal rotation (turning your thighs inward)

>> Adduction (bring your legs inward, like when you cross your knees)

>> Hip flexion (forward folds or even child's pose — especially flexion with abduction and adduction, such as pigeon)

You should also probably avoid the poses such as the following:

>> Standing forward bend (hip flexion and internal rotation — it should be okay after you're fully healed or if you limit how far you bend forward by placing your hands on your thighs)

>> Child's pose (hip flexion)

>> Eagle (hip flexion and adduction)

>> Cow face (hip flexion and adduction)

Knee Replacements

Like all joints in the human body, the knees are subject to routine wear, damage, or even disease. The primary reason someone would want to either partially or completely replace a knee joint is to alleviate the constant pain associated with degeneration, to restore the ability to move normally, or very often both.

The most common cause of a knee joint failure is:

>> Osteoarthritis

>> Rheumatoid arthritis

>> Injury

Note: For more information on dealing with arthritis, see Chapter 16.

Types of knee replacements

Two primary surgical approaches deal with the knees:

>> Partial knee replacement

>> Total knee replacement

A partial knee replacement is more straightforward than a complete replacement (though the results often don't last as long). This procedure

>> Is performed on an out-patient basis

>> Targets only one side of the knee

>> Typically requires less bone to be removed

>> Leads to quicker recovery time

>> Requires easier rehab after surgery

>> Presents a lower risk of infection

Partial knee replacements are usually done on people who have issues with just one area of the knee. The surgery is less complicated, and you have a greater probability of regaining natural movement.

A *total knee replacement,* on the other hand, involves replacing a complete knee joint. This procedure

>> Is performed on an in-patient basis

>> Requires more time to perform than partial knee replacement (surgery usually takes one to four hours)

>> Creates often scar tissue (which may impact mobility)

Yoga and knee replacements

Yoga can offer people with knee replacements some specific benefits by:

>> Strengthening the muscles that surround and support the knees (including the muscles that support the new knee joint)

>> Rediscovering a sense of balance

>> Enhancing mobility that may have been lacking prior to surgery or developed after the surgery

Yoga offers so many other health benefits that people often want to return to Yoga as soon as possible. Your doctor or physical therapist will give you important guidance in that regard.

It will be important for you to keep in mind three critical questions:

>> How much pain is still present?

>> How long has it been since your surgery?

>> How long has it been since you completed your physical therapy?

To keep your new joint safe (regardless of what kind of surgery you had), you need to avoid going to extremes in terms of your range of motion. Too much twisting can certainly be damaging.

Keep the following suggestions for safety in mind:

>> **Your toes should track with your knees.** Or, said another way, make sure that your toes are pointing in the same direction that your knees are moving.

>> **Stack your joints.** In many standing poses, I ask you to keep your knees above your ankle joints. This, I believe, not only gives you more stability, but it also eliminates the injury risks associated with having your knees too far in front of your feet (so that you can't see your toes).

>> **Come out of any pose that seems to put strain on your knees.** You can always revisit a pose once your knee gets stronger and more flexible.

TIP

Kneeling is often uncomfortable (but not damaging) on artificial knees (especially using a thin mat on a hardwood floor or stone tile). You can often alleviate the discomfort by doubling or rolling part of the mat under the knees or using some kind of cushion, such as a folded blanket.

Poses to make you wary

Certain Yoga postures (especially some of the standing poses) can help build up the surrounding muscles that support the knees. The only thing you need to do is remember the suggestions for safety I mention in the preceding section.

Certain poses, however, put too much twist or pressure on the knee joint and should be avoided:

>> Pigeon

>> Hero's (sitting back between your feet)

>> Thunderbolt (sitting back on your heels)

>> Full (low) squat to the heels

>> Eagle wrap

>> Lotus

Even simple poses like child's pose or happy baby may require the knees to bend beyond a comfortable range. While you can certainly make modifications to any of these poses, I recommend that you just leave them out.

Chapter **15**

Boning Up on Osteoporosis

As you get older, your doctor may talk to you about the risks of osteoporosis — and for good reason. This disease can cause your bones to weaken so much that even a little stumble and fall can cause a serious fracture (most often in your hip, spine, or wrist).

Loren Fishman, MD, my friend and author of the book, *Yoga for Osteoporosis: The Complete Guide* (2010), has done some pioneering research that suggests Yoga can help limit the disease in the first place. Or, if you've already been diagnosed with diminished bone density, he talks about how Yoga may be able to help you, as well.

But recent medical research also points to the fracture-risks associated with doing certain Yoga postures, and it's certainly a matter of debate within the medical community just how much Yoga can help. That's why it's so important that you talk with your own healthcare providers — and, if you practice Yoga, work with a teacher — ideally, a Yoga therapist — who knows all about the condition in the first place.

Bone strength is usually at its highest in your 20s. Bone is living tissue and, simply stated, a constant process takes place in your body where old bone is broken down and new bone replaces it. The problem, as you get older, occurs when the creation of new bone doesn't keep up with the loss of old bone.

Who Gets Osteoporosis

About 80 percent of people who get osteoporosis are women. So yes, women are more likely to get the disease. But men need to be aware that they, too, can get it. According to the National Osteoporosis Foundation, one in two women and up to one in four men over age 50 will break a bone due to osteoporosis. Additionally, a man is more likely to sustain a fracture due to osteoporosis than he is of developing prostate cancer. While anyone can get osteoporosis, certain people are more at risk:

>> Caucasian and Asian women

>> Older people — especially women (post-menopausal)

>> People with a family history of the disease

>> People with smaller frames

>> People whose hormone levels are out of balance

>> Anyone who does not consume enough calcium

Osteoporosis Symptoms

Unfortunately, often people with osteoporosis don't find out they have the disease until their first bone fracture. That's why I want to encourage you to talk with your healthcare provider.

The only sure way to determine the strength of your bones is to have them tested with a bone mineral density test. It is noninvasive and painless and can reveal critical information, either good or not so good.

Your bone density can be compromised, but still not be in the range of osteoporosis. In some cases, you may be heading toward the disease, and your bone strength is diminished enough for you to be diagnosed with *osteopenia.*

People with osteopenia are not at as high a risk of a fracture as someone with osteoporosis. Still, people with osteopenia must take into account their weakened bone density. But hold on; this condition is complex. That's why you need a specialist in osteoporosis on your team.

Yoga and Osteoporosis

You've probably seen a variety of commercials that talk about the various drugs that are available to treat osteoporosis. You should talk to your doctor and weigh the benefits versus risks of the medications themselves. A calcium-rich diet and perhaps calcium supplements with vitamin D, which helps you absorb calcium, may also be prescribed.

Doctors often recommend exercise as well, perhaps strength training, weight-bearing aerobic activities, and flexibility, stability, and balance exercises. Here's how Yoga can fit into your regime.

While Yoga can be a great way to help either prevent osteoporosis or address the problem of reduced bone density, it is critically important to practice safely. And, just like with medication, you should begin to treat an existing problem — regardless of the approach — only under the guidance of your medical professional.

Hinging from the hips versus bending from the waist

REMEMBER

The following advice is probably important to anyone who practices Yoga if the goal is better health and fitness: Hinge from the hips and do NOT bend from the waist. The difference between the two movements may at first seem subtle, but the distinction is actually huge.

Just as you can with the other joints I cover in this book, you can use your spine in good and not-so-good ways. To safely fold forward (whether you're doing a Yoga pose or picking up socks off the floor), the action needs to take place in your hip joints — a structure that's designed to hinge forward and back (see Figure 15-1).

On most people, the waist falls somewhere between the bottom of your rib cage and the top of your navel (see Figure 15-2). If you trace that around, you're probably somewhere in the area of your lumbar spine. If you try to bend from there, you can move as far as your vertebrae want to move and then you begin to put stress on both your lower and mid-spine. For those people diagnosed with osteoporosis in the spine, this stress may be enough to cause a fracture.

REMEMBER

As you consider how Yoga can help build bone density, keep in mind that any movement requiring extreme spinal flexion (bending forward) can cause compression that may potentially lead to some kind of fracture.

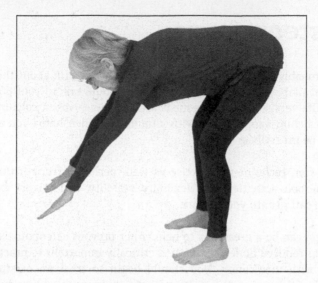

FIGURE 15-1:
Hinging from the hips.

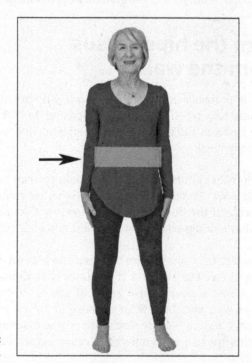

FIGURE 15-2:
The waist.

WARNING

Be extra careful or avoid the following types of movements altogether:

>> Rolling up from a standing forward fold

>> Yoga bicycles

>> Twisting poses (especially while bending forward because these movements can compress your spine)

>> Pigeon pose or other hip openers

>> Adjustments from teachers trying to stretch you out

Yoga routine for bone health

When dealing with osteoporosis and osteopenia, the biggest concern is how vulnerable you are to fractures. You should talk to your doctor or other healthcare provider about where Yoga might fit in to your routine.

With that in mind, the following Yoga sequence may be good for you, starting with chest-to-belly breathing. This breathing technique gently opens or externally rotates the spine, which is good for both osteoporosis and osteopenia.

1. **Start in a comfortable standing position (see Figure 15-3).**

2. **Inhale while expanding the chest from the top down and continuing this movement downward into the belly; pause for a couple seconds.**

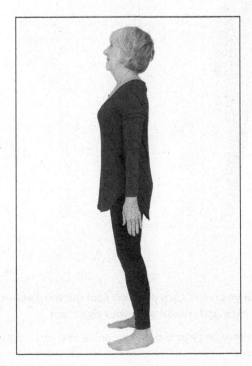

FIGURE 15-3: Chest-to-belly breathing.

3. **Exhale while gently contracting and drawing the belly inward, starting just below the navel; pause for a couple seconds.**

4. **Repeat 6 to 12 times.**

Arm raises with a head turn can gently extend (straighten) your upper back:

1. **Stand tall with your arms at your side.**

2. **As you inhale, bring your right arm up until it is reaching over your head (your elbow can be slightly soft) and turn your head to the left.**

3. **Exhale as you lower your arm and turn your head back to center.**

4. **Repeat four to five times on each side, alternating arms (see Figure 15-4).**

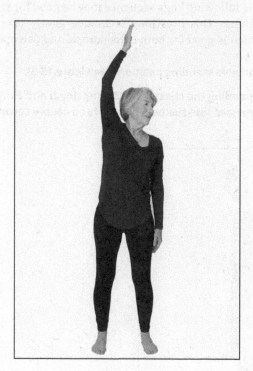

FIGURE 15-4:
Alternating arm raises.

Warrior I:

1. **From the back of your mat, turn your left foot outward about a quarter turn and take a big step forward with your right foot.**

   Your right knee should be directly over your ankle, and your thigh should be parallel to the floor.

2. Place your hands on your hips and square your hips forward.

3. Keep both legs straight and hang your arms at your sides in the ready position.

4. As you inhale, raise your arms forward and overhead; at the same time bend your right knee to a right angle (see Figure 15-5).

   You should feel like you're in a classic runner's stretch, with a light pull in your left calf.

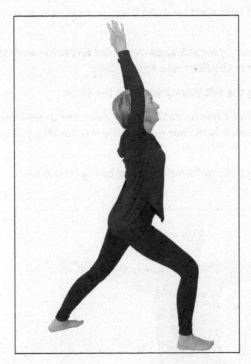

FIGURE 15-5:
Warrior I.

5. As you exhale, straighten your right leg and bring your arms back to the ready position as in Step 1.

6. Repeat three times and then hold the pose for about 30 seconds (five to seven breaths).

7. Step out of the pose and repeat on the left side

Warrior II:

1. Turn sideways on your mat, as you exhale, step out to the right about 3 to 3 1/2 feet with your right foot.

2. Turn your left foot out 90 degrees and your right foot 45 degrees.

   An imaginary line drawn from your right heel toward your left foot should bisect the arch of your left foot.

3. Face forward and as you inhale, raise your arms out to the sides parallel to the line of the shoulders (and the floor) so that your arms form a T with the torso.

4. As you exhale, bend your left knee over your left ankle so that your shin is perpendicular to the floor (see Figure 15-6).

5. If possible, bring the left thigh parallel to the floor.

6. Repeat Steps 3 and 4 two more times (for a total of three), keeping your arms in a T, and then turn your head to the left, looking out over your left fingertips.

7. Stay for six to eight breaths before going to the next pose.

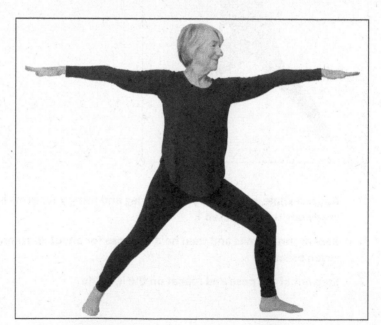

FIGURE 15-6:
Warrior II.

Extended side angle:

1. From your warrior II pose, shift your torso sideways, extending your left arm along side your left ear.

2. As you inhale, stand up straight again.

3. Repeat two more times, keeping your shoulders level as you lean out; hold this position and breathe.

4. On an exhalation, bring your left arm all the way to your left knee, bending the arm and resting it on the knee; at the same time, bring the right arm up and overhead (along the side of your ear), reaching forward (see Figure 15-7).

5. Hold this position for four to six breaths and then return to the previous pose.

6. Do both warrior II and the extended side angle pose on the other side.

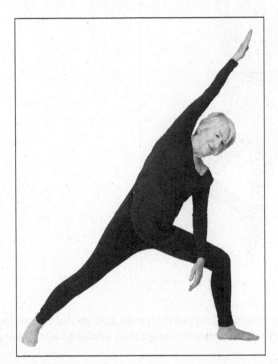

FIGURE 15-7:
Extended side angle pose.

Tree pose:

1. **Stand tall on your mat.**

2. **As you exhale, place the sole of your left foot on the inside of your right leg — above or below your knee — toes pointing toward the ground (see Figure 15-8).**

3. **As you inhale, bring your arms overhead and join your palms together; look at a spot on the floor six to eight feet in front of you.**

4. **Hold for six to eight breaths and then repeat on the other side.**

   If needed, you can put one of your hands on the wall for support.

TIP

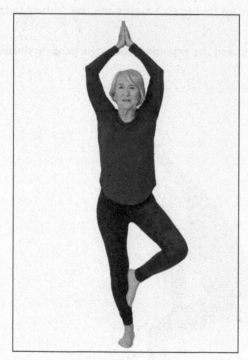

FIGURE 15-8:
Tree pose.

If you have been diagnosed with osteopenia and you're not as likely to sustain a fracture, you may want to try a variation that I refer to as the karate kid pose:

1. **Stand tall on your mat.**

2. **As you inhale, raise your arms out to the sides in a T, not higher than your shoulders.**

3. **Focus on a spot on the floor six to eight feet in front of you.**

4. As you exhale, bend your right knee, lifting it toward your chest (see Figure 15-9).

5. Hold for six to eight breaths.

6. Repeat with your left knee.

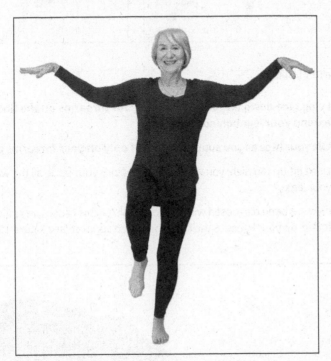

FIGURE 15-9: Karate kid.

Balancing cat:

1. Beginning on your hands and knees, position your hands directly under your shoulders with your palms down, your fingers spread on the floor, and your knees directly under your hips. Straighten your arms, but don't lock your elbows.

2. As you exhale, slide your left hand forward and your right leg back, keeping your hand and your toes on the floor.

3. As you inhale, raise your left arm and right leg to a comfortable height (see Figure 15-10).

   If you're unable to hold this pose, skip Step 3.

WARNING

4. Hold for four to five breaths.

5. Repeat on the other side.

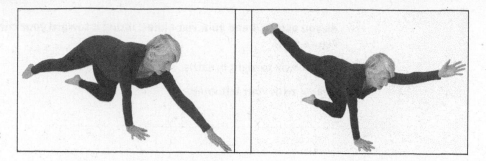

FIGURE 15-10:
Balancing cat.

Forearm plank:

1. **Lying face-down on your mat, place your forearms on the floor and extend your legs behind you.**

2. **Lift your hips as you support yourself only on your forearms and toes.**

   Don't lift up too high; you want a flat line from your back, all the way down to your legs.

   If you've been diagnosed with osteoporosis or this causes any pain or discomfort, drop your knees to the floor for added support (see Figure 15-11).

WARNING

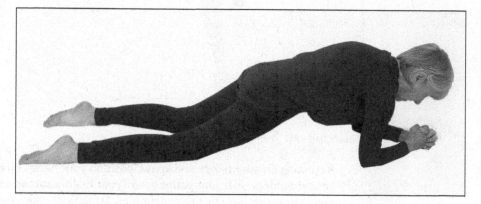

FIGURE 15-11:
Plank pose (with modification).

Locust variation:

1. **Lie flat on your belly with a folded blanket under your hips.**

2. **Place your legs at hip width with the front of your feet on the floor.**

3. **Rest your forehead on the floor and your arms on the floor, along the sides of your body, palms down.**

4. **As you inhale, raise your chest, head, and right leg (see Figure 15-12).**

TIP

If the pose is too strenuous, try just bending the leg at the knee. For an even easier variation, raise your chest without lifting your leg at all.

5. **As you exhale, lower your trunk, head, and leg slowly back to the floor.**
6. **Repeat six to eight times.**
7. **Repeat on the other side.**

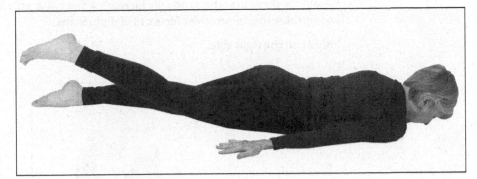

FIGURE 15-12:
Locust pose.

Prone corpse:

If you're completing this sequence, then you're already on your stomach. Place your hands underneath your forehead (like a pillow) and just rest (see Figure 15-13).

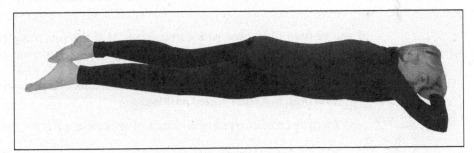

FIGURE 15-13:
Prone corpse.

Seated twists:

1. **Sit flat on the floor, with a folded blanket or a cushion to raise your hips, your legs extended in front of you at hip width.**
2. **Bend your left knee and place the left foot on the floor with the heel near your groin and four to six inches from your right thigh.**

3. Place your left palm on the floor behind you, near your tailbone; turn your fingers away from your hips.

4. Bend your right arm and place your right elbow outside of your left knee with your fingers pointing up.

5. As you inhale, lift your chest and head, bringing your back up nice and tall (see Figure 15-14).

6. As you exhale, rotate your shoulders and upper back to the left.

7. Repeat for three breaths, gradually increasing the twist; stay in your comfortable maximum twist for six to eight breaths.

8. Repeat on the right side.

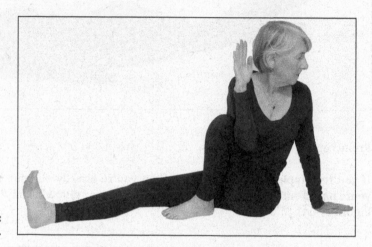

FIGURE 15-14:
Seated twist.

If you've been diagnosed with osteoporosis or if the preceding twisting posture causes any pain, consider doing the following variation instead:

1. Sit tall on your mat, with several folded blankets or a cushion to raise your hips, in a cross-legged position.

   For more comfort, try siting on a stack of blankets or a cushion to raise your hips.

   One blanket isn't usually enough!

TIP

2. As you inhale, place your left hand flat on the floor behind you and your right hand on your left knee.

3. As you exhale, move deeper into the twist while looking over your left shoulder (see Figure 15-15).

4. Hold the pose for five breaths (perhaps sitting taller on each inhalation and twisting deeper on each exhalation) and then switch to the other side.

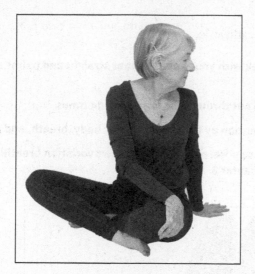

FIGURE 15-15:
Seated twist
variation.

Reclined arm raises:

1. **Lie flat on your back with your arms at your sides, palms down.**

2. **As you inhale, slowly raise your right arm up and overhead (touching the floor behind you, if possible) and turn your head to the left (see Figure 15-16).**

3. **As you exhale, bring your arm back to your side and bring your head back to the center.**

4. **As you inhale, slowly raise your left arm up and overhead (touching the floor behind you, if possible) and turn your head to the right.**

5. **As you exhale, bring your arm back to your side and bring your head back to the center.**

6. **Repeat the arm raise four to six times on each side.**

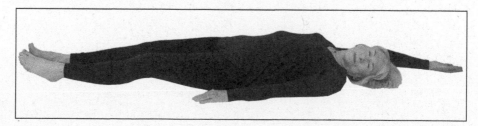

FIGURE 15-16:
Reclined arm
raises.

Corpse pose with breathwork:

1. Lie on your back with your knees bent or straight and palms up (see Figure 15-17).

2. Breathe in and out through the nose 12 to 14 times.

3. Focus your attention by trying to link your body, breath, and mind.

4. Staying in corpse pose, perform the bellows variation breathing exercise described in Chapter 3.

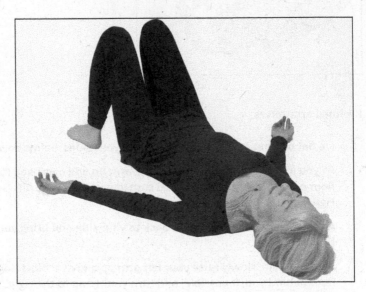

FIGURE 15-17: Corpse pose.

Chapter **16**

Handling Arthritis

Probably no one condition is more associated with growing older than arthritis, although younger people can suffer from the condition too.

Arthritis is a catchall term to refer to joint pain or joint disease. And as the symptoms of arthritis get more severe — stiffness, swelling, decreased range of motion — your daily activities become more and more challenging to accomplish.

The good news? In many studies, Yoga is shown to help. In this chapter, I review some of the most common types of the condition and describe ways in which you can use Yoga to possibly prevent or reduce arthritis symptoms.

What Is Arthritis?

Arthritis can take many forms. It may refer to any one of the following:

» Osteoarthritis (or degenerative joint disease)

» Rheumatoid arthritis

» Infectious arthritis

» Other arthritic conditions (including ankylosing spondylitis, bone spurs, gout, and systemic lupus)

Only your doctor can tell you if you're suffering from any of these forms of arthritis. While each of these conditions is unique, their symptoms may be similar.

Common symptoms

The most common symptoms of arthritis involve joint pain or swelling. Depending on the type of arthritis diagnosed by your doctor, your symptoms may include

>> Pain

>> Stiffness

>> Swelling

>> Redness

>> Decreased range of motion

Contributing factors

While this chapter is not intended to help you self-diagnose any type of arthritis, you should be aware of factors that may contribute to its development:

>> **Age:** Arthritis occurs more frequently as people age. And certain types of arthritis tend to get worse with age.

>> **Family history:** While you may not have inherited a fortune from a rich relative, your arthritis may be inherited from your family. Certain types of arthritis can be passed along from one generation to the next.

>> **Obesity:** Here's yet another reason to keep your weight down: Excess pounds tend to put additional stress on the joints. It's not surprising then that overweight people are more prone to developing arthritis.

>> **Gender:** While arthritis seems to be an equal opportunity offender, statistically speaking, women are more likely to develop rheumatoid arthritis, while men are more likely to suffer from gout.

>> **Previous injuries to a joint:** It's truly a case of adding insult to injury: If you did sustain some kind of joint damage (say, for example, a sprained ankle), you may be more likely to develop arthritis in that joint.

Osteoarthritis and Rheumatoid Arthritis

Osteoarthritis and rheumatoid arthritis are the most common types of arthritis:

» *Osteoarthritis,* which can be quite painful, is a degenerative joint disease (usually found in the weight-bearing areas of the body: the hips, knees, neck, lower back, or hands). It often develops in injured joints or joints that have sustained a lot of stress from use or even from too much weight. Cartilage gets thinner or disappears altogether, causing bone-on-bone friction. The joints often become less flexible and can even swell or develop bone spurs.

» *Rheumatoid arthritis* is an inflammatory disease involving the autoimmune system. It's often found in the smaller joints of the hands, wrists, elbows, shoulders, knees, ankles, and feet. The problem with autoimmune diseases is that they cause the production of certain enzymes that attack healthy tissue, including joint linings. Rheumatoid arthritis can also cause intense pain, swelling, lack of mobility, and even deformities. Rheumatoid arthritis leads to fatigue, fever, unintended weight loss, inflammation of the eyes, anemia, bumps beneath the skin, or even lung inflammation.

Discovering How Yoga Can Help

While osteoarthritis and rheumatoid arthritis are two distinct forms of the disease, Yoga may help to address both through

» Pain management

» Improved flexibility and range of motion

» Balancing of the immune system

» Weight loss

» Cardio improvement

» Reduced stress

It would be negligent of me not to point out that certain foods can be both good and bad for arthritis. Aside from general improvements to your health (especially in the areas of weight and heart health) associated with a thoughtful diet, certain foods may be inflammatory. This inflammation can leading to increased symptoms for the type of arthritis that's associated with your autoimmune system.

REMEMBER

Nutrition advice should not come from your Yoga teacher or Yoga therapist — unless he or she also has training and credentials in diet. Rather, talk to your doctor or to a trained nutritionist about the best diet for you — especially if you're dealing with inflammatory arthritis.

What Yoga can help you with, however, is gentle stretching and strengthening, as well as some breath work, which may help to prevent the disease in the first place, or deal with the symptoms — especially stress.

A Joint-Freeing Routine for Home

The following sequence is based on an ancient routine from India that was popularized in the United States by the late Mukunda Stiles. It is a series of movements designed to bring flexibility to all the major joints.

If you're trying to keep your joints arthritis-free, this sequence is great for general joint health. If you're currently dealing with arthritis symptoms, this routine may provide you with some relief and even increase mobility.

REMEMBER

As always, pay attention to how your body is feeling. If any particular movement causes you pain, please modify it so it feels right or skip it entirely. And pay particular attention if you've had any joint replacements because certain movements may not be your friend. (See Chapter 14 on dealing with joint replacements.)

Start sitting on a stack of blankets or bolster with your legs extended in front of you. (You can also do this routine in a chair if getting on the floor is too challenging.)

1. As you exhale, flex your feet (pull your toes back toward you).

2. As you inhale, point your feet (see Figure 16-1).

3. Repeat for a total of six to eight times.

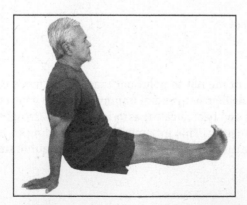

FIGURE 16-1:
Point and flex
your feet.

Soles together:

1. **Bring your feet together with your big toes touching.**

2. **As you inhale, flip your feet, connecting the soles (see Figure 16-2).**

3. **As you exhale, return your feet back to the starting position.**

4. **Repeat for a total of six to eight times.**

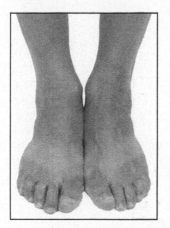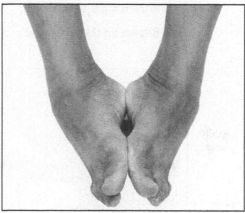

FIGURE 16-2:
Soles together.

Rotate your feet:

1. **Rotate your feet (circle your ankles).**

2. **Rotate your feet to the right (circle your ankles).**

3. **Repeat for a total of six to eight times.**

4. **Repeat in the opposite direction (see Figure 16-3).**

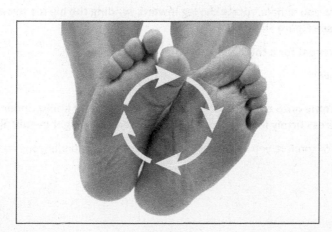

FIGURE 16-3:
Rotate your feet.

Bend and straighten your leg:

1. Bend your left leg, placing the sole of the foot flat on the floor and keeping the right leg as straight as possible.

2. Clasp your hands behind the left calf.

3. As you inhale, extend your left leg as straight as possible (see Figure 16-4).

4. As you exhale, bend the leg and return your foot to the floor.

5. Repeat eight times total.

6. Repeat on the other side.

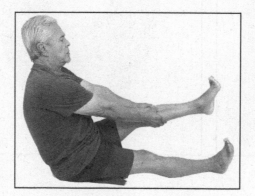

FIGURE 16-4:
Bend and straighten your leg.

Rotate your leg:

1. Sitting tall, separate your legs into a V-shape.

2. As you inhale, rotate the right leg outward, sending the pinky toe toward the ground.

3. As you exhale, rotate the leg inward, sending the big toe toward the floor (see Figure 16-5).

4. Repeat for a total of eight times.

Cat/cow:

1. Come onto all-fours, wrists under shoulders and knees under hips, and press firmly into the hands, fingers wide and weight evenly distributed.

   For comfort, you may want to put a folded blanket under your knees.

WARNING

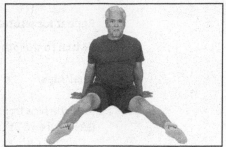

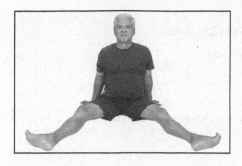

FIGURE 16-5:
Rotate your leg.

2. As you exhale, round your back like a cat with your head down.

3. As you inhale, arch your lower back like a cow and look up.

4. Repeat for a total of eight times (see Figure 16-6).

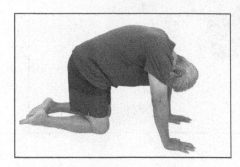

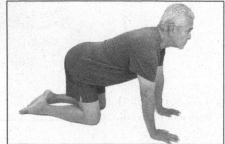

FIGURE 16-6:
Cat/cow routine.

Cat/cow variation:

1. As you inhale, extend LEFT leg straight behind you and look up.

2. As you exhale, bring your knee toward your forehead, slightly rounding your back (see Figure 16-7).

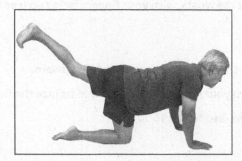

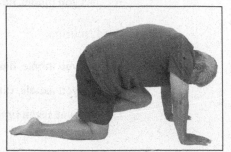

FIGURE 16-7:
Cat/cow variation.

3. **Repeat for a total of eight times.**

4. **Switch to the other side.**

Rock your hips:

1. Rock the hips from side to side, inhaling to one side and exhaling to the other (see Figure 16-8).

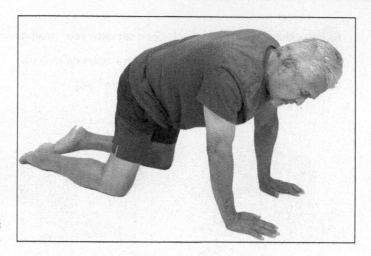

FIGURE 16-8:
Rock your hips.

Wrist flex:

1. **Move into a seated position, cross-legged, if possible.**

   If needed, you can sit on a stack of folded blankets or a chair.

2. **Extend your arms parallel to the floor in front of you, fingers straight out.**

3. **As you exhale, send your fingers toward the floor, bending your wrists.**

4. **As you inhale, flex the wrists, with your fingers facing up (see Figure 16-9).**

Wrist routine:

1. **As you inhale, flip the wrists so your palms face upward.**

2. **As you exhale, turn your hands over so your palms face the floor.**

3. **Repeat seven times (see Figure 16-10).**

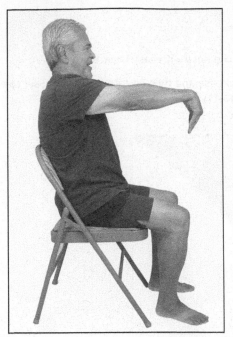 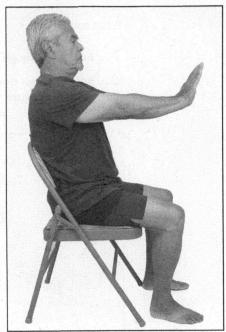

FIGURE 16-9:
Wrist flex.

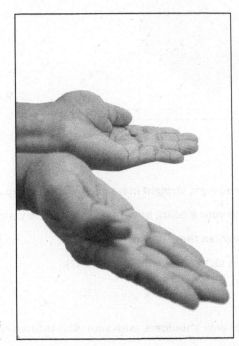

FIGURE 16-10:
Wrist routine.

Wrist rotation:

1. Breathe through the nose with easy breath.

2. Rotate wrists clockwise and then counter-clockwise, six to eight times each (see Figure 16-11).

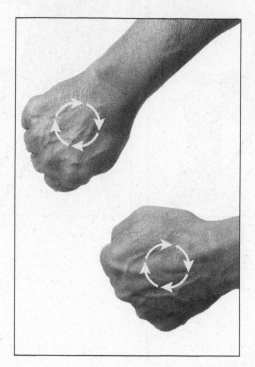

FIGURE 16-11:
Wrist rotation.

Elbow routine:

1. As you inhale, extend arms straight in front of you, palms up.

2. As you exhale, bend your elbows, bringing your hands to your shoulders.

3. As you inhale, straighten them back out.

4. Repeat for a total of eight times (see Figure 16-12).

Shoulder routine:

1. Bring your hands to your shoulders, with your elbows forward.

2. As you inhale, open your elbows out to the sides (see Figure 16-13).

3. As you exhale, connect the elbows at center.

4. Repeat for a total of eight times.

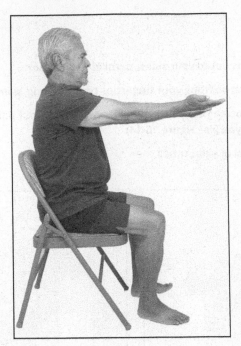
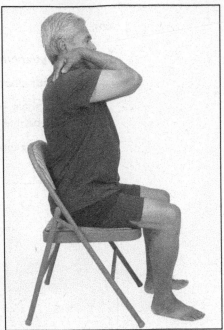

FIGURE 16-12:
Elbow routine.

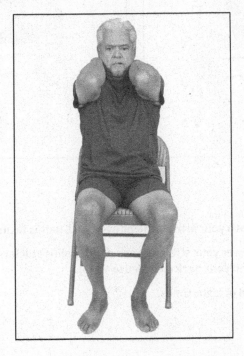
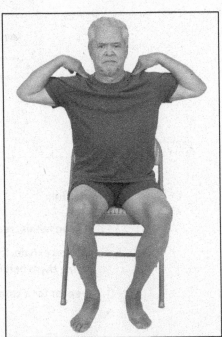

FIGURE 16-13:
Shoulder
rotation.

Arm rotation:

1. Extend your arms out to your sides, parallel to the floor.

2. Bend your elbows pointing your fingertips to the ceiling, palms forward.

3. As you exhale, rotate your arms downward, sending your palms toward the wall behind you (see Figure 16-14).

4. Repeat for a total of eight times.

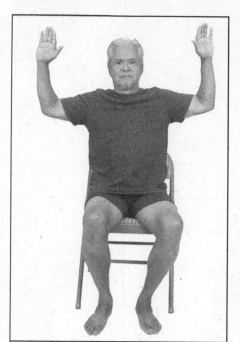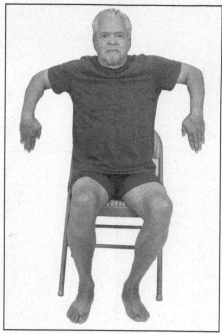

FIGURE 16-14:
Arm rotation.

Arm routine:

1. On an inhale, reach your arms straight overhead, palms facing.

2. As you exhale, lower your straight arms down, palms still facing, and bring them behind your back (see Figure 16-15).

3. Repeat for a total of eight times.

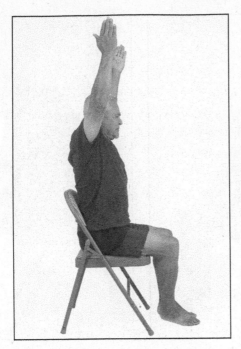 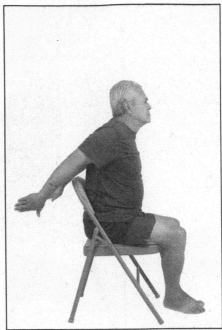

FIGURE 16-15:
Arm routine.

Seated cat/cow:

1. Sit on your chair with your hands on your knees.

2. As you inhale, arch the back, squeeze the shoulder blades together, and look up.

3. As you exhale, round the back forward and look down (see Figure 16-16).

4. Repeat for a total of eight times.

Seated side bend:

1. As you exhale, hang your right hand toward the floor and gently bend to right.

2. Inhale back to the center (see Figure 16-17).

3. Repeat for a total of six to eight times.

4. Switch to the other side.

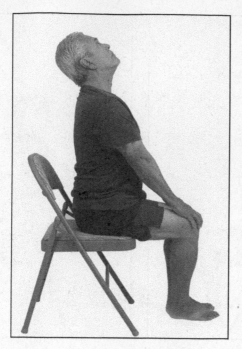
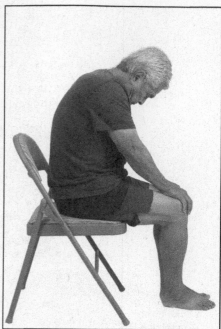

FIGURE 16-16: Seated cat/cow.

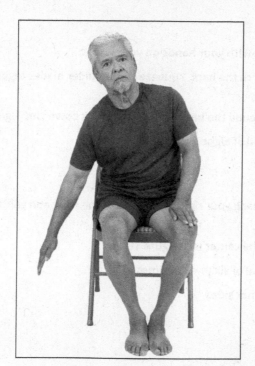

FIGURE 16-17: Seated side bend.

Seated twist:

1. Inhale and sit up tall.

2. Grasp your right knee with your left hand; put your left hand on the back of the chair.

3. As you exhale, twist to the right, keeping your spine long. (See Figure 16-18.)

4. As you inhale, come back to center.

5. Repeat for a total of eight times.

6. Twist to the other side.

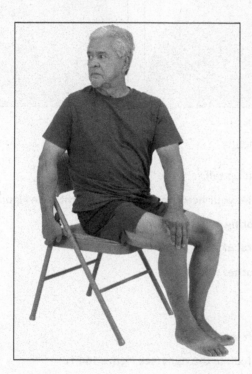

FIGURE 16-18: Seated twist.

Neck extension/flexion:

1. Inhale, sending your head gently back, only as far as feels comfortable for you.

2. Exhale, lower your chin to your chest.

3. Repeat for a total of six to eight times (see Figure 16-19).

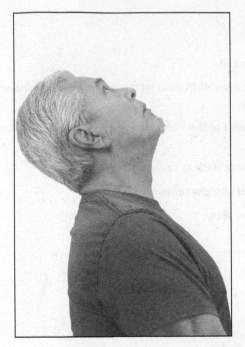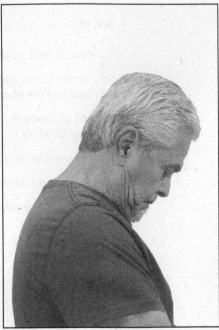

FIGURE 16-19:
Neck flexion.

Lateral neck movement:

1. **On an inhale, sit up tall.**

2. **As you exhale, let your head tip gently to the right. (See Figure 16-20.)**

3. **As you inhale, bring your head back to center.**

4. **Repeat for a total of six to eight times.**

5. **Repeat on the other side.**

Neck rotation:

1. **On an inhale, sit up tall.**

2. **As you exhale, look to the right (see Figure 16-21).**

3. **As you inhale, come back to center.**

4. **Repeat for a total of six to eight times.**

5. **Repeat on the other side.**

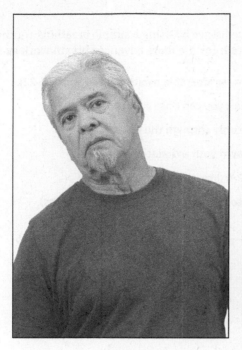

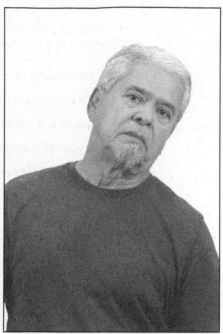

FIGURE 16-20:
Lateral neck
movement.

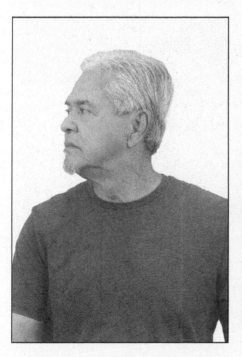

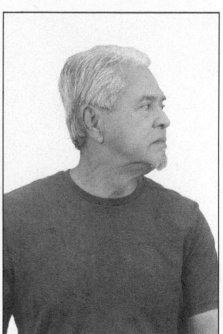

FIGURE 16-21:
Neck rotation.

Finally, complete this sequence by doing a simple breathing routine as outlined in Chapter 3 as a preparation for the more advanced breath work exercises.

TIP

1. **Continue to sit in a comfortable position (see Figure 16-22).**

   If it helps you to relax, you can close your eyes.

2. **Inhale and exhale only through the nose.**

3. **If you can, slow down your exhalation.**

   Make your exhalation take longer than your inhalation.

4. **Continue for one to two minutes (eight to ten breaths).**

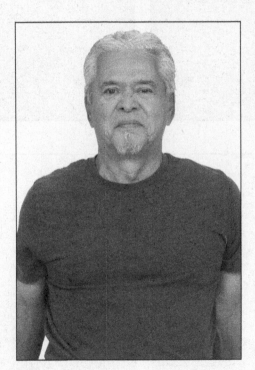

FIGURE 16-22:
Easy breath work.

Chapter **17**

Understanding Menopause and Andropause

Many people over 50 have started to experience changes in hormone levels that indicate the onset of menopause in women and andropause in men. Both of these natural phases of life need to be understood and managed — and once again, Yoga can help!

Some people may experience this time of transition as physically and emotionally challenging, while others are able to smoothly navigate through it, finding a new sense of freedom with the physiological changes that naturally occur during this time of life. In some cultures, these changes are honored, appreciated, and even celebrated, representing a shift from one phase of life to another.

Hormonal Changes in Women and Men

For women, menopause is probably more well known, and perhaps slightly more anticipated. *Menopause* is the point in a woman's life when ovaries stop producing eggs and the body reduces the amounts of estrogen and progesterone that it produces.

For men, while reproductive capabilities are not necessrily halted, andropause is a decline in the production of those hormones that help in the reproductive process, particularly androgen and testosterone.

Menopause

Menopause is a natural phase of life for women, characterized foremost by the end of the menstrual cycle (monthly periods). While women typically experience this phase somewhere between 40 and 60, the most common time is the early fifties.

Signs that menopause is nearing (called *perimenopause*) include:

>> Irregular periods

>> Hot flashes

>> Night sweats or chills

>> Mood fluctuations

>> Unexplained weight increases

Other symptoms may potentially arise, so women need to continue seeing their doctor or gynecologist to monitor their health.

While menopause generally occurs naturally, with age, other things may bring it on at any age:

>> Total hysterectomy

>> Chemotherapy or radiation

>> Problems when ovaries aren't functioning properly

Post-menopause

REMEMBER

Yoga is not intended to be a substitute for your regular medical resources. If you think you are going through menopause or post-menopause and have concerns, talk with your doctor. Because of decreased hormone production, women in menopause may be more susceptible to osteoporosis and possibly various heart complications.

Andropause

Equating andropause in men to menopause in women may seem somewhat inappropriate. Menopause is a much more prominent condition and represents more profound biological changes.

Andropause may, in fact, be more appropriately called age-related testosterone deficiency. Signs that you may have a testosterone deficiency include:

>> Sexual problems

>> Memory or concentration problems

>> Weight gain or loss of muscle mass

>> Trouble sleeping

>> Reduced self-confidence or depression

If you are symptomatic, your doctor may suggest some kind of testosterone replacement therapy. Along with some measurable benefits with this approach, unfortunately, just like with hormone replacement therapy for women, there are a number of serious risks. You need to have your testosterone level checked first and then discuss with your doctor the best way to move forward.

Breath Work at Home: Cooling Breath

Cooling breath is a general breathing technique that is even mentioned in Yoga texts written centuries ago. Traditional Yoga believes that this breathing technique reduces body temperature, relieves stress, decreases thirst, and increases the level of moisture throughout the body.

While breath work can be a beneficial exercise for anyone, it is often particularly recommended to women dealing with hot flashes.

1. **Sit in a comfortable Yoga posture on the floor or on a chair and relax your body**

2. **Curl your tongue lengthwise and let its tip protrude from your mouth, as shown in Figure 17-1.**

3. **Slowly suck in air through the tube formed by your tongue and exhale gently through the nose.**

4. **Repeat this breath 10 to 15 times.**

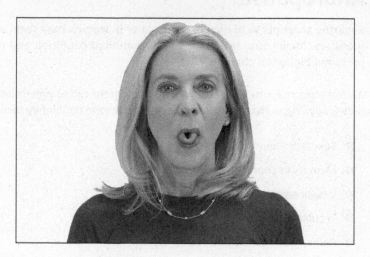

FIGURE 17-1:
Cooling breath.

If you can't curl your tongue (an ability determined by your genes — seriously!), you can practice the crow's beak technique instead. Using this technique, you pucker your lips (like you're drinking through a straw), leaving just enough space for the air to pass through (see Figure 17-2). Again, you inhale through your mouth and exhale through your nose.

A third option for doing this breathing technique is using what's called the hissing breath:

1. **Slowly extend your tongue between your teeth, allowing your lips to widen like a smile.**

2. **As you inhale, allow your breath to pass over the sides of your tongue, making a hissing sound.**

3. **At the top of the inhalation, draw the tongue in and close the mouth.**

4. **Slowly exhale through the nostrils only (see Figure 17-3).**

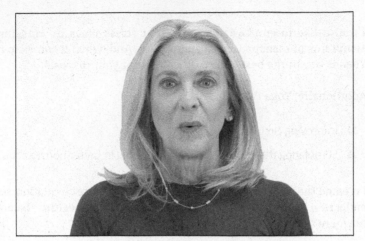

FIGURE 17-2:
Crow's beak
technique.

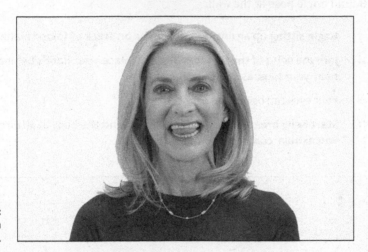

FIGURE 17-3:
Hissing breath
technique.

Yoga at Home

Yoga can help transform what can be a challenging time of your life into a more enjoyable journey. Indeed, not only can Yoga help relieve some of the physical and emotional symptoms associated with hormonal changes; it can also help increase your overall strength and flexibility.

In terms of mood swings associated with hormonal changes, it is worth noting that Yoga releases *endorphins* — hormones that make you feel good. Yoga can also reduce the production of stress hormones, such as cortisol. The ultimate effect can help promote a state of wellness in your body and help encourage both physical and mental healing.

I'd also like to emphasize the role that stress plays in worsening some of the symptoms of menopause and andropause. And, when it comes to reducing stress, Yoga is one of the best tools that's readily at your disposal.

Additionally, Yoga can help with

>> Improving circulation

>> Stimulating the endocrine system (resulting in better hormone balance)

I created the following home routine to help promote circulation and stimulate the endocrine system, which in turn encourages a healthy, balanced release of hormones.

Bound angle pose at the wall:

1. **Begin sitting up against a wall, maybe on stack of folded blankets.**

2. **Join the soles of the feet together and place your hands behind your legs, near your hips, as shown in Figure 17-4.**

   Your eyes can be opened or closed.

3. **Start belly breathing (as you inhale, expand the belly in all directions; as you exhale, contract and release).**

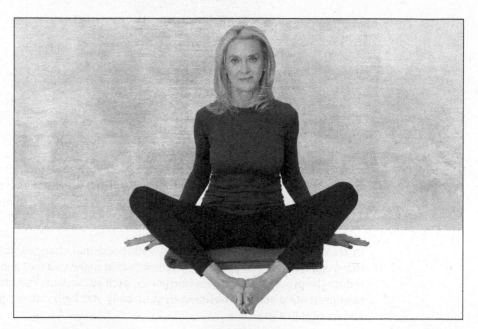

FIGURE 17-4:
Bound ankle pose at the wall.

Wide angle pose at the wall:

1. **Still sitting at the wall, widen your legs out to a comfortable position (continue with the belly breathing).**

   You can choose whether you want to have your feet and ankles relaxed or tilted back toward you (see Figure 17-5).

2. **Hold for eight to ten breaths.**

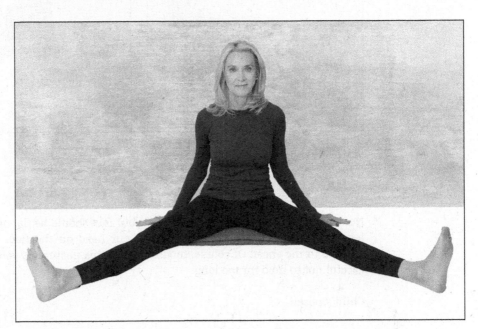

FIGURE 17-5:
Wide angle pose
at the wall.

Downward facing dog:

1. **Start on your hands and knees; straighten your arms, but don't lock your elbows (see Figure 17-6a).**

   Be sure that the heels of your hands are directly under your shoulders, palms on the floor, fingers spread, and your knees directly under your hips.

2. **As you exhale, lift and straighten (but don't lock) your knees; as your hips lift, bring your head to a neutral position so that your ears are between your arms.**

3. **Press your heels toward the floor and your head toward your feet, as in Figure 17-6b.**

Don't complete this step if doing so strains your neck.

4. **Repeat Steps 1 through 3 two more times (for a total of three times) and then stay in Step 3 for six to eight breaths.**

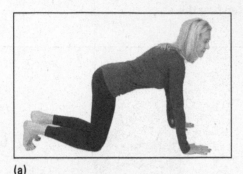

(a)

FIGURE 17-6A:
On all fours with straight arms.

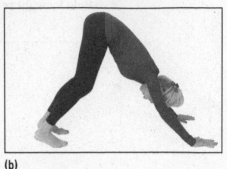

(b)

FIGURE 17-6B:
Downward facing dog.

Note: In the classic form of this posture, your feet should be flat on the floor, your legs and arms straight, and the top of your head on the floor with your chin pressed to the chest. Of course, modify any of this posture as you need to and be careful not to hold for too long.

Child's pose:

1. **Starting on your hands and knees, place your knees about hip width apart with your hands just below your shoulders.**

You want your elbows straight but not locked.

2. **As you exhale, sit back on your heels; rest your torso on your thighs and your forehead on the floor.**

You don't have to sit all the way back.

3. **Lay your arms back on the floor beside your torso with your palms up or reach your relaxed arms forward with your palms on the floor.**

If it's more comfortable, you can spread your knees and let your torso fall in between.

TIP

4. **Close your eyes and stay in the folded position for six to eight breaths (see Figure 17-7).**

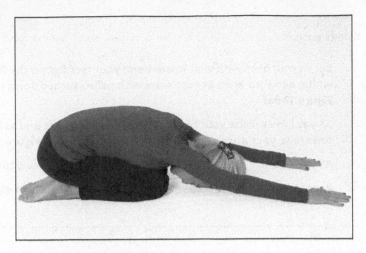

FIGURE 17-7:
Child's pose.

Supported child's pose:

1. Sitting back with your knees spread wide, pull a bolster between your legs, near your groin.

2. Bend forward and come to rest on the bolster (see Figure 17-8).

TIP

Feel free to experiment with comfort. If you don't have a bolster, try a stack of folded blankets or perhaps a bed pillow. Even if you do have a bolster, make sure it's built up enough to be comfortable.

3. Try different positions with your arms and find the position that is most comfortable.

4. Continue with belly breathing, staying in this position long enough to relax.

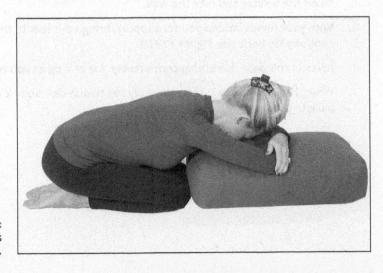

FIGURE 17-8:
Supported child's
pose.

Bridge pose:

1. Lie on your back with your knees bent, your feet flat on the floor at hip width, and your arms at your sides with palms turned down (see Figure 17-9a).

2. As you inhale, raise your hips to a comfortable height and at the same time raise your arms overhead to touch the floor (see Figure 17-9b).

3. As you exhale, return your hips to the floor and your arms to your sides.

4. Repeat Steps 3 and 4 six to seven more times (for a total of eight).

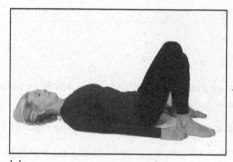

(a)

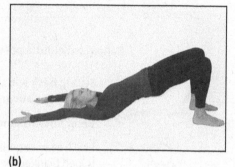

(b)

FIGURE 17-9A: Bridge setup.

FIGURE 17-9B: Bridge with arm Lift.

Feet on the wall:

1. Place a bolster about 3 feet from a wall.

2. Sit on the bolster and face the wall.

3. With your hands behind you for support, bring your feet to the wall and carefully lay back (see Figure 17-10).

4. Relax in this pose, breathing comfortably, for as long as you want.

5. When you're ready to get up, carefully roll to one side and sit with your back to the wall.

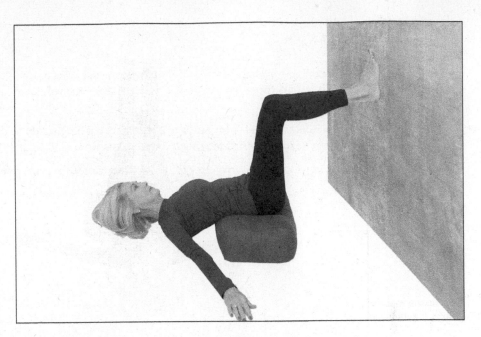

FIGURE 17-10:
Feet on the wall.

Legs up the wall with variations:

1. Sit on a bolster close to the wall, sideways.

2. Swing your legs up the wall, moving in as close as you can.

3. Bring the soles of your feet together, making a diamond-shaped, bound angle pose against the wall (see Figure 17-11).

4. Hold and breathe for about ten breaths (still trying to maintain that belly breath).

5. Straighten your legs and then let them go wide into a split (see Figure 17-12).

6. Hold for ten more easy breaths.

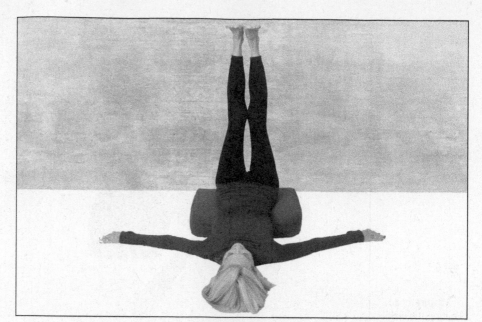

FIGURE 17-11:
Legs up the wall,
soles together.

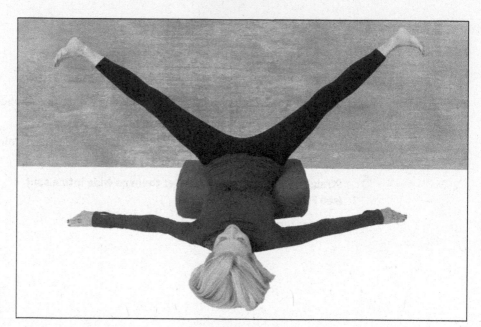

FIGURE 17-12:
Legs up the
wall, split.

Twisting pose:

1. **Lie on your back with your knees bent and feet on the floor at hip width.**

2. **Extend your arms out from your sides like a T (in line with the top of your shoulders) with your palms down.**

3. **As you exhale, slowly lower your bent legs to the right side while turning your head to the left (see Figure 17-13).**

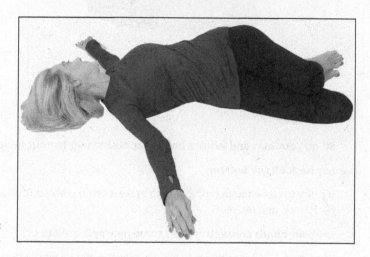

FIGURE 17-13:
Twisting pose.

4. **Turn your head the opposite direction of your legs.**

5. **Hold for six to eight breaths.**

6. **As you inhale, bring your bent knees back to the middle.**

7. **Repeat on the other side.**

Knees to chest variation:

1. **Lie on your back and bend your knees in toward your chest.**

2. **Hold your kneecaps (see Figure 17-14).**

3. **Begin circling your knees in on direction for four to six times.**

4. **Reverse the direction for four to six times.**

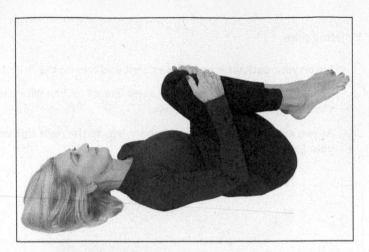

FIGURE 17-14:
Twisting pose.

Supported corpse posture:

TIP

1. **Sit on your mat and bring a bolster or cushion up to your lower back.**

2. **Lay back on the bolster.**

   Be sure to use enough cushioning to make it completely comfortable on your back, neck, and head.

3. **Let your hands come to rest on some nearby blankets.**

   See Figure 17-15 for this setup. It's actually one of my favorite positions to be in, but feel free to make any adjustments you would like, based on your own personal comfort and the props you have on hand.

4. **Allow your mind and body to completely relax, continuing to breathe only through your nose (if possible).**

   Stay for as long as you would like.

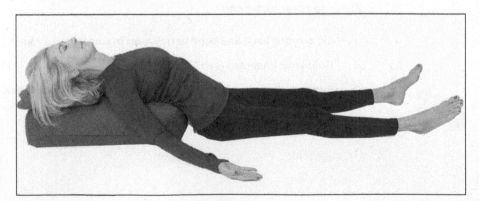

FIGURE 17-15:
Supported
corpse pose.

Chapter **18**

Helping the Pelvic Floor

You may have heard people talk about their pelvic floors, although that muscle group is certainly less prominent than some of other muscles. Unlike the rippled abdominals you see at the beach or the leg muscles that help you walk or run, most of the muscles of the pelvic floor are located deep inside you, and their function tends to be of a more personal nature, which can make them more challenging to discuss.

Both Women and Men Have Pelvic Floors

Of course, both women and men have pelvic floors. As the name suggests, the *pelvic floor* consists of a group of muscles that span across the bottom of the pelvis, from the tailbone to the two sit bones to the side-walls of the pelvis to the pubic bone in the front. The pelvic floor also includes the urethral and anal sphincter muscles that we use to control bowel and bladder functions.

One of the many jobs of the pelvic floor is to provide support to certain organs that are common to both genders: the bladder and bowel. Women, however, also have pelvic organs that are involved in pregnancy and giving birth: the uterus, cervix, and vagina. These organs in many ways can make the female pelvic floor and its function even more complicated.

Making a Move

One of the most basic aspects of the pelvic floor muscles is that they need to move. As your diaphragm descends into your abdominal cavity every time you inhale, so, too, does your pelvic floor move and stretch. Your pelvic floor muscles also move when:

>> **Going to the bathroom:** When you tighten the pelvic floor muscles, you're essentially preventing your bladder and bowel from releasing anything. Conversely, relaxing those same muscles opens the doors.

>> **Performing sexual functions:** The ability to relax and engage the pelvic floor muscles contributes to sexual health in both men and women.

>> **Having babies (during pregnancy, delivery, and after):** In women, pelvic floor health is an essential part of pre- and post-natal care. These muscles need to be relaxed during delivery and also need to be able to be engaged in functional ways pre- and post-natal. Sometimes vaginal deliveries can damage these muscles, and pelvic rehabilitation with a pelvic floor health professional can help.

>> **Maintaining spinal health:** Because the spine is an area of the body that's of particular interest to me, I want to mention that the pelvic floor muscles play a role in spinal health by their coordinated movement in timing with the breath, as well as other muscles that support the spine.

>> **Controlling balance:** Believe it or not, the pelvic floor also plays a role in your ability to maintain balance and avoid falling! The pelvic floor moves in time with your breath and with other core muscles that contribute to balance. Holding or contracting the pelvic floor muscles too tightly can interrupt the body's natural strategies to balance and prevent falls.

Like most of the muscle movements in your body, pelvic floor muscle movement can become more limited or restricted. Indeed, those muscles can become so tight that they're ultimately incapable of doing their job.

The good news is, like most of the muscles in your body, the pelvic floor can be exercised. My objective in this chapter is simply to make you aware of this muscle group and give you some Yogic approaches to keeping it flexible and to keeping things moving.

Knowing When to See a Doctor

As you get older, your body changes and may not function in the same way it used to function. Of course, I believe that Yoga in general can help you maintain a healthy body (and mind). Still, I would never suggest that Yoga can be a substitute for your doctor. I strongly encourage you to seek medical attention if you think this area of your body is malfunctioning.

Some pelvic floor symptoms that may indicate problems include:

>> Chronic constipation

>> Urgency to urinate

>> Frequent urination

>> Urinary or bowel leakage

>> Pain:

- Genital or rectal

- Pelvis area

- Back (especially lower back)

- Hip or groin

- During sexual arousal, intercourse, erection, or orgasm

- During urination or defecation

Although some of these issues may be common, they're actually a sign of some dysfunction in the system, and you can do things to prevent or address them. While medical science is always trying to gain deeper insight into the causes of these problems, the truth is many issues are complex, and often a combination of multiple factors contribute to whether a problem emerges.

The following are some of the potential risk factors with pelvic floor issues:

>> Age

>> Obesity

>> Pregnancy/childbirth (for women)

>> Straining when going to the bathroom

>> Coughing (especially chronic)

>> Lifting heavy things

>> Rigorous exercise

Additional risk factors include:

>> Excessive pelvic floor muscle tension

>> Unmanaged stress and anxiety

>> Sensitized nervous system

>> Past experience of persistent pain

>> Adverse childhood experiences or trauma

>> Certain abdominal or pelvic surgeries

You have control over some of these things, but not others. You can, however, consciously address many factors that contribute to keeping the pelvic floor muscles healthy, flexible, and mobile. And that's precisely where Yoga comes in.

Yoga and the Pelvic Floor

As you may guess, many Yoga practices may help with the engagement, relaxation, and movement of the pelvic floor muscles in timing with the breath, keeping them strong and flexible, and helping them to relax when necessary. I suggest that Yoga can help enhance pelvic floor health in many different ways, incidentally or not. For your home routine, however, I would like to suggest a more direct approach.

Yoga has specific techniques known as *bandhas*, a Sanskrit word that can be translated to mean *locks*. I commonly think of three:

>> Contraction of the anal sphincter *(anal lock)*

>> Contraction of the stomach muscles, into the rib cage *(belly lock)*

>> Tucking the chin into the chest *(chin lock)*

When it comes to anal locks, experts disagree on exactly which of the pelvic floor muscles should be engaged: the actual anal sphincter muscles, deep perineum muscles, vaginal muscles, or all the muscles of the pelvic floor. Some Yoga experts suggest that anal locks and Kegel exercises are one and the same, while others argue that they're completely different. I'll let your doctor settle that one for you.

And while the debate may be interesting, one of my colleagues pointed out that almost no one can totally isolate specific muscles in the pelvic floor, anyway. If this point is true, the distinction may be insignificant.

Home Yoga Routine for the Pelvic Floor

Yoga experts are more than happy to tell you when and how the lock techniques described in the preceding section should be performed. Unfortunately, the experts don't always agree.

I certainly don't want to drag you into a debate that, while important, is often a bit esoteric. Instead, I simply share with you a technique that one of my teachers in India said I should practice every day.

WARNING

This routine is intended to strengthen and mobilize your pelvic floor muscles (as well as others). It is not intended to cure problems you may already have. In fact, these locks could even exacerbate certain problems, so if you're having issues, please see your healthcare provider first.

REMEMBER

Your pelvic floor muscles need to move; they need to contract (tighten) and they need to relax. So, the relaxation portion of this routine is just as important as the tightening.

This technique requires the use of two locks, involving both the anal sphincter and the abdominal muscles.

1. **Find a comfortable, reclined position and, if it feels okay on your back, straighten your legs (see Figure 18-1).**

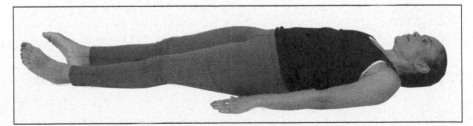

FIGURE 18-1:
Finding a
comfortable
position.

2. **Take three or four deep breaths, inhaling and exhaling through the nose, if possible.**

3. **Inhale and then exhale all the air out of your body.**

4. **With the air still out, tighten your anal sphincter and pull your abdominal muscles inward.**

   Your stomach will completely flatten and may even collapse as you pull your navel back toward your spine. Your pelvis will probably tip toward upward (see Figure 18-2).

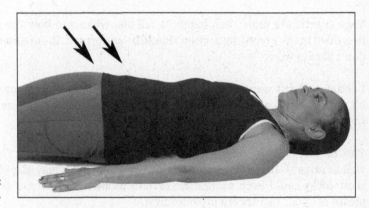

5. **Hold for three to five seconds.**

6. **Exhale completely, relaxing your anal sphincter and abdominal muscles.**

7. **Repeat this sequence up to ten times.**

WARNING

While I've been safely doing and teaching this routine for over 30 years, I still strongly recommend that, if you have high blood pressure or may be at risk for a stroke or heart attack, you should skip this routine entirely. Instead, talk to your doctor or cardiologist to see if this type of exercise is appropriate.

5
Routines for Home

Learn three unique Yoga routines to do when you have only 5 minutes.

Discover three Yoga routines for when you have 15 minutes. Exploring three Yoga routines for when you have 30 minutes.

Chapter **19**

Five-Minute Routines for Home

I f you have only five minutes to practice, this chapter contains three routine options. I have given these sequences a lot of consideration, especially because it's such a limited period of time.

What You Need to Know

In each pose, I provide you with the steps to get into the pose, but I may also point you to other places in this book that talk about a certain pose.

REMEMBER

It may take you additional time to complete the sequence as you read the instructions next to each pose. The sequence will go much quicker once you learn how to get into each pose.

Finally, if a particular pose seems too challenging or causes pain, modify it in a way that works for you or skip it entirely. Knowing what's good for your body and what isn't is truly a sign of being an advanced Yoga practitioner.

Routine 1

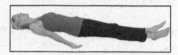

Corpse pose

1. Lie flat on your back, with your arms stretched out and relaxed by your sides, palms up (or whatever feels most comfortable). You can Place a small pillow or folded blanket under your head and another large one under your knees for added comfort. Bend your knees if it feels better on your back.

Inhale and exhale only through your nose (unless you have a cold or allergies or some other reason your nasal passages are blocked). Take 8 to 12 breaths. (Try the Belly breathing technique with a long exhale described in Chapter 3.)

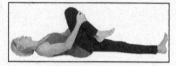

Knee to chest

2. Lie on your back with both legs straight. As you exhale, draw one knee into your chest and hold on to it with both hands, just below the knee cap. Bring your toes back toward you. Stay for six to eight breaths. (Keep the other leg straight or place your foot on the ground with your knee bent if it feels better on your back.) *Note:* If you are having knee problems, you can use both hands to hold underneath the knee.

Repeat with the other leg.

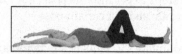

Bent leg arm raise

3. Lie on your back with one leg bent and one leg straight. Start with your arms at your side, palms down. As you inhale, bring both arms overhead. As you exhale, bring your arms back to your sides. Repeat two more times.

Next, on an inhalation, bring both arms overhead again, but this time keep your arms overhead as you exhale and then inhale. Try to stretch your arms even further. On your next exhalation, bring your arms back down. Do the same sequence on the other side.

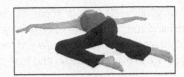
Windshield wiper

4. Lie on your back with both knees bent and feet on the ground, wide apart. Your arms are at your sides, palms down. As you exhale, drop both knees to the right. As you inhale, bring both knees back up. As you exhale, let both knees fall to the left.

Repeat three times on each side and then stay on the right for four to five breaths. Repeat, leaving your knees down on the other side.

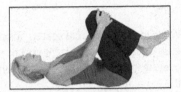
Knee to chest

5. Lie on your back and bend your knees in toward your chest. Hold your shins just below the knees. If you have any knee problems, hold the backs of your thighs instead.

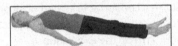
Corpse with left nostril breathing

6. Lie on your back with your knees bent or straight, feet on the ground, and palms up. Breathe in and out through the nose, 4 to 6 times. Try to be in the moment, linking your body, breath, and mind.

Use your right thumb to gently block off your right nostril. Breathe in and out through just the left nostril for 12 to 15 slow breaths. (For more information on left nostril breathing, see Chapter 3.)

Routine 2

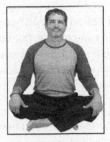
Easy pose

1. Sit on your mat with your legs straight out in front of you and place your hands on the floor beside your hips with your palms down and fingers pointing forward. Shake your legs up and down a few times to get the kinks out.

Bend your knees and cross your ankles in front of you, sitting comfortably.

Rest your hands on your knees with your arms relaxed and palms down. Lengthen your spine by stretching your back in an upward motion, balance your head over your torso, and look straight ahead.

Stay for six to eight breaths, using Focus breathing (see Chapter 3).

Note: To help you sit straighter and lessen the strain on your back, sit on a bolster or folded blanket.

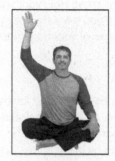

The single arm raise

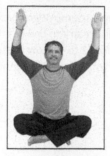

Arm raises

2. While in a comfortable seated position (stay in easy pose), raise your right arm from the front over head on an inhalation; lower your arm on the exhalation.

Still in a comfortable seated position, raise your left arm on your next inhalation; lower your arm on the exhalation.

Raise both arms (like in the photo) from the front overhead on your next inhalation; lower both arms on the exhalation.

Repeat this sequence one time.

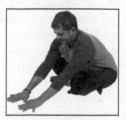

Seated cross-legged forward bend

3. Still in your seated position (easy pose), take a big inhale. As you exhale, put both hands in front of you on your mat (palms down) and slide out as far as your body wants to go. Inhale back up.

Repeat two more times and hold the stretch for four to six breaths.

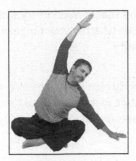

Seated side bend

4. Continue sitting comfortably in a cross-legged position. Place your left palm on the floor, near your left hip.

As you inhale, raise your right arm out to the side and up above your head beside your right ear. As you exhale, slide your left hand across the floor out to the left, letting your torso, head, and right arm follow as you bend to the left. *Note:* Don't let your buttocks come off the floor as you bend.

Inhale back to the upright position. Repeat two more times and hold the stretch for four to six breaths.

Repeat on the other side.

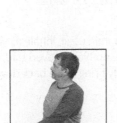

Seated twist

5. Still in a comfortable cross-legged position, place your left hand palm down on top of your right knee. Put your right hand down behind your right hip.

As you inhale, extend your spine upward. As you exhale, twist your torso and head to the right.

Repeat this movement for two more breaths, gradually twisting farther with each exhalation, but don't force it. Hold the twist for six to eight breaths.

Repeat on the other side.

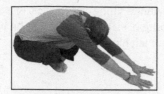

Seated cross-legged
forward bend

6. From this seated position, try sliding forward just to see whether your range of motion has increased.

Hold the stretch for four to six breaths. Finish the routine in the seated position, taking 8 to 10 breaths (using Focus breathing).

Routine 3

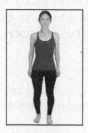

Mountain pose
(with chest-to-
Belly breathing)

1. Stand tall but relaxed with your feet at hip width; hang your arms at your sides, palms turned toward your legs. Visualize a vertical line connecting your ear, your shoulder, and the sides of your hip, knee, and ankle.

While in this pose, employ the chest-to-Belly breathing technique described in Chapter 3, taking six to eight breaths.

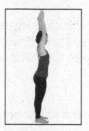

Standing arm
raises

2. Still in mountain pose, inhale as you slowly raise both arms overhead, from the front. Slowly bring them back down as you exhale.

Keeping your tall posture, repeat this movement four to six more times.

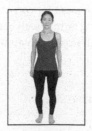

Rejuvenation
sequence

3. Stand in the mountain posture with your feet at hip width and arms at your sides.

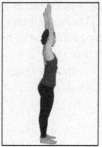

Rejuvenation
sequence

As you inhale, slowly raise your arms out from the sides and up overhead.

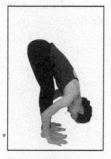

Rejuvenation
sequence

As you exhale, bend forward from the waist and bring your head toward your knees and your hands forward and down toward the floor in the standing forward bend.

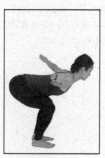

Rejuvenation
sequence

Bend your knees quite a bit and as you inhale, sweep your arms out from the sides, but only come halfway up with your arms in a T (half forward bend).

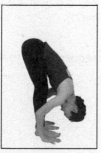

Rejuvenation
sequence

As you exhale, fold all the way down again and hang your arms in the standing forward bend.

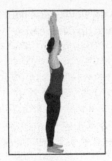

Rejuvenation
sequence

As you inhale, sweep your arms from the sides like wings and bring your torso all the way up again, standing with your arms overhead in the standing arm raise.

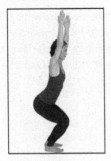

Rejuvenation
sequence

As you exhale, bend your knees and squat halfway to the floor.

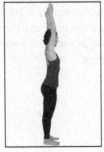

Rejuvenation
sequence

As you inhale, bring your torso all the way up again, standing with your arms overhead in the standing arm raise.

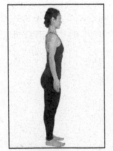

Rejuvenation
sequence

As you exhale, bring your arms back to your sides as in Step 1.

Repeat this sequence four to six times.

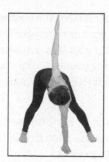

Standing twist

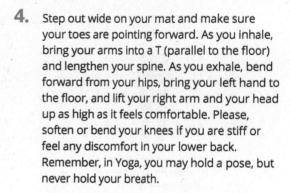

4. Step out wide on your mat and make sure your toes are pointing forward. As you inhale, bring your arms into a T (parallel to the floor) and lengthen your spine. As you exhale, bend forward from your hips, bring your left hand to the floor, and lift your right arm and your head up as high as it feels comfortable. Please, soften or bend your knees if you are stiff or feel any discomfort in your lower back. Remember, in Yoga, you may hold a pose, but never hold your breath.

As you inhale, return to the starting position. Repeat this movement on the same side and, on the third time, hold your left hand down and your right hand reaching up. Your head can be looking up, in the middle, or down. Stay for four to six breaths. If you want to make it more challenging, move your left hand, which is on the ground, closer to your right foot.

After holding for four to six breaths, repeat the same sequence on the other side.

5. Still folding forward, come back to the middle, bringing your hands to the floor for support or maybe clasping the opposite elbow.

Stay for four to five breaths.

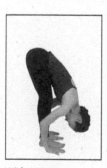

Wide stance
forward fold

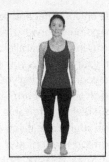

Mountain pose (with chest-to-Belly breath)

6. Stand tall but relaxed with your feet at hip width; hang your arms at your sides, palms turned toward your legs. Visualize a vertical line connecting your ear, your shoulder, and the sides of your hip, knee, and ankle.

While in this pose, perform the chest-to-Belly breathing exercise described in Chapter 3. Try to do 10 to 15 breaths.

Chapter **20**

Fifteen-Minute Routines for Home

If you have only 15 minutes to practice, this chapter contains three routines for you. I have given these sequences a lot of consideration, oftentimes using postures to both compensate for a pose that occurred before and prepare your body for a posture that's coming up.

In each pose, I provide you with the steps to get into the pose, but I also point you to other places in this book that talk about a certain pose.

It may take you additional time to complete the sequence as you read the instructions next to each pose. The sequence will go much quicker once you learn how to get into each pose.

Finally, if a particular pose seems too challenging or causes pain, modify it in a way that works for you or skip it entirely. Knowing what's good for your body and what isn't is truly a sign of being an advanced Yoga practitioner.

Routine 1

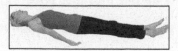

Corpse pose with Focus breathing

1. Lie flat on your back, with your arms stretched out and relaxed by your sides, palms up (or whatever feels most comfortable). Place a small pillow or folded blanket under your head and another large one under your knees for added comfort. Bend your knees if it feels better on your back. (You can review Focus breathing in Chapter 3.)

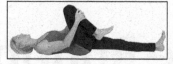

Knee to chest

2. Lie on your back with both legs straight. As you exhale, draw one knee into your chest and hold on with both hands, just below the knee cap. Bring your toes back toward you. Stay for six to eight breaths. (Keep the other leg straight or place your foot on the ground with your knee bent if it feels better on your back.)

Note: If you're having knee problems, you can use both hands to hold underneath the knee.

Repeat on the other side.

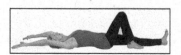

Bent leg arm raise

3. Lie on your back with one leg bent and one leg straight. Start with your arms at your side, palms down. As you inhale, bring both arms overhead. As you exhale, bring your arms back to your sides. Repeat two more times.

On an inhalation, bring both arms overhead again, but this time keep your arms overhead as you exhale and then inhale, trying to stretch your arms even further. On your next exhalation, bring your arms back down. Repeat. Do the same sequence on the other side.

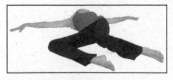

Windshield wiper

4. Lie on your back, both knees bent and feet on the ground, wide apart. Your arms are at your sides, palms down. As you exhale, drop both knees to the right. As you inhale, bring both knees back up. As you exhale, let both knees fall to the left.

Repeat three times on each side and then stay on the right for four to six breaths. Repeat, leaving your knees down on the other side for four to six breaths.

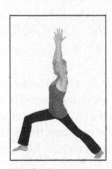

Warrior I

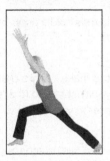

variation 1

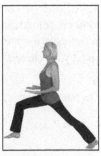

variation 2

5. Stand in the mountain posture and as you exhale, step forward approximately 3 to 3.5 feet (or the length of one leg) with your right foot.

Your left foot turns out naturally, but if you need more stability, turn it out more (so that your toes point to the left).

Place your hands on the top of your hips and square the front of your pelvis; release your hands, and hang your arms. Bend your forward knee. If you can't see your toes, step out further. Then, straighten your front leg and hang your arms.

As you inhale, raise your arms forward and overhead and bend your right knee to a right angle (so that the knee is directly over the ankle and the thigh is parallel to the floor).

If your lower back is uncomfortable, lean the torso slightly over the forward leg until you feel a release of tension in your back (see the first variation).

As you exhale, return to the starting place; soften your arms and face your palms toward each other, looking straight ahead. Repeat three times and then stay for four to six breaths.

Bring your arms down, parallel to the floor, and pull your elbows back while extending your hands forward (palms up). As you pull your shoulder blades closer together, it may help to imagine you're holding a tray (see the second variation). Stay for four to six breaths.

Repeat on the other side.

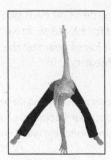

Standing twist

6. Step out wide on your mat and make sure your toes are pointing forward. As you inhale, bring your hands to your hips and lengthen your spine. As you exhale, bend from your hips, draw your stomach in, and fold forward. (Keep your knees soft or bent if you feel any discomfort in your lower back.) Place your hands on the mat.

Moving your right hand underneath your face, reach your left hand upward from the side on your next inhalation. Exhale as you bring your arm back down. Repeat this twisting movement (on the same side) for a total of three times and then hold.

REMEMBER

In Yoga, you may hold a pose, but never hold your breath.

If you want to make it more challenging, you can move your right hand (that's on the ground) closer to your left foot.

Hold for four to five breaths and repeat on the other side.

7. Still folding forward, come back to the middle, bringing your hands to the floor for support or perhaps clasping your elbows.

Stay for four to five breaths.

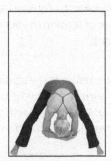

Wide stance
forward fold

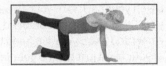

Balancing cat

8. Beginning on your hands and knees, position your hands directly under your shoulders with your palms down, your fingers spread on the floor, and your knees directly under your hips. Straighten your arms, but don't lock your elbows.

As you exhale, slide your right hand forward and your left leg back, keeping your hand and your toes on the floor. As you inhale, raise your right arm and left leg to a comfortable height.

Hold for four to six breaths; repeat on the other side.

To challenge yourself, you can move the extended arm and leg side to side slowly.

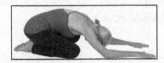

Child's pose

9. Starting on your hands and knees, place your knees about hip width apart with your hands just below your shoulders. You want your elbows straight but not locked.

As you exhale, sit back on your heels; rest your torso on your thighs and your forehead on the floor. You don't have to sit all the way back.

Close your eyes and stay in the folded position for six to eight breaths. (If this is uncomfortable, you can either place blankets or a bolster under your chest, or you can lie on your back with your knees pulled into your chest.)

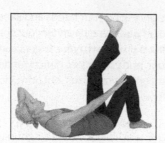

Slide ups

10. Lie on your back with your knees bent and your feet flat on the floor. Bend your left elbow and place your left hand on the back of your head just behind your left ear.

Raise the left leg as close to vertical (90 degrees) as possible, but keep your knee slightly bent. Draw the top of your foot toward your shin to flex your ankle and place your right palm on your right thigh near your pelvis. As you exhale, sit up slowly halfway and slide your right hand toward your knee.

Keep your left elbow back in line with your shoulder and look at the ceiling. Don't throw your head forward.

Repeat this movement four more times and then switch to the other side. (If you want extra support for your neck, use both hands behind your head.)

Note: If you want to make it more challenging, stay up for an extra breath before coming back down.

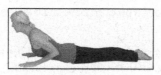

Cobra

11. Lie on your belly with your thumbs near your armpits, fingers forward and head down. As you inhale, pull forward and up, like a turtle coming out of a shell. Keep your buttocks loose. Repeat six to eight times.

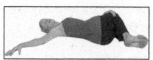

Reclined bent leg twist

12. Lie on your back with your knees bent and your feet on the ground. Bring your arms out into a T with the palms down.

As you exhale, drop both bent knees to the left. As you inhale, bring them both up. Repeat three times and on the third time, stay down for six to eight breaths. Repeat on the other side.

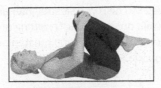

Knees to chest

13. Lie on your back and slowly bring your knees in toward your chest to tolerance. If you have knee problems, you can hold under your thighs. Stay for six to eight breaths.

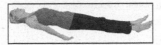

Corpse with left nostril breathing

14. Staying in corpse pose, use your right thumb to gently block off your right nostril. Breathe in and out through just the left nostril for 12 to 15 breaths.

For more information on left nostril breathing, see Chapter 3.

Routine 2

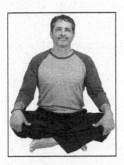

Easy pose

1. Sit on your mat with your legs straight out in front of you and place your hands on the floor beside your hips with your palms down and fingers pointing forward. Shake your legs up and down a few times to get the kinks out.

Bend your knees and cross your ankles in front of you, sitting comfortably.

Rest your hands on your knees with your arms relaxed and palms down. Lengthen your spine by stretching your back in an upward motion, balance your head over your torso, and look straight ahead.

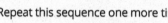

Note: To help you sit straighter and lessen the strain on your back, try sitting on a bolster or stack of blankets for all seated poses in this routine.

Stay for six to eight breaths, using the Focus breathing technique in Chapter 3.

2. While in a comfortable seated position (stay in easy pose), raise your right arm from the front over head on an inhalation; lower your arm on the exhalation.

Raise your left arm on your next inhalation; lower your arm on the exhalation.

Raise both arms overhead on your next inhalation; lower both arms on the exhalation.

Repeat this sequence one more time.

Arm raises

Arm raises

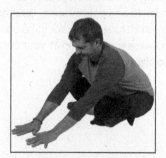

Seated cross-legged forward bend

3. Still in your seated position (easy pose), take a big inhale. As you exhale, put both hands in front of you on your mat (palms down) and slide your arms out as far as your body wants to go. Inhale as you sit back up.

Repeat two more times and hold the stretch forward for four to six breaths.

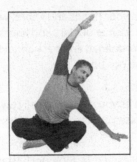

Seated side bend

4. Continue sitting comfortably in a cross-legged position. Place your left palm on the floor, near your left hip.

As you inhale, raise your right arm out to the side and up above your head beside your right ear. As you exhale, slide your left hand across the floor out to the left, letting your torso, head, and right arm follow as you bend to the right.

Note: Don't let your buttocks come off the floor as you bend.

Inhale back to the upright position. Repeat two more times and hold the stretch for three to five breaths.

Repeat on the other side.

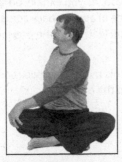

Seated twist

5. Still in a comfortable cross-legged position, place your left hand palm down on top of your right knee. Put your right hand down on the floor behind your right hip.

As you inhale, extend your spine upward. As you exhale, twist your torso and head to the right.

Repeat this movement for two more breaths, gradually twisting farther with each exhalation (don't force it). Hold the twist for six to eight breaths.

Repeat on the other side.

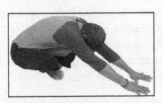

Seated cross-legged forward bend

6. From this seated position, try sliding forward to see whether your range of motion has increased.

Again, hold the stretch for four to six breaths.

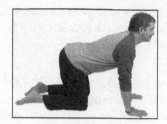

Cow pose

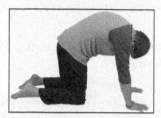

Cat pose

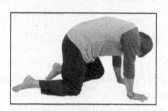

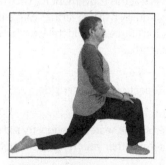

Cat-cow variation

7. Get on your hands and knees, with your wrists under your shoulders and knees under your hips. Your head and back should be in a neutral position.

Inhale as you drop your belly toward the mat and raise your chin upward (this is cow pose).

As you exhale, draw your chest inward and round your back upward. You are now looking downward, bringing your chin toward your chest (this is cat pose).

Repeat this movement two more times.

8. Still on your hands and knees, bring your chin toward the ceiling as you inhale, at the same time lifting and extending your left leg out behind you. As you exhale, bring your leg and bent knee in as your back comes into the cat poses you learned in the previous step.

Repeat this movement two more times, then switch to the other side.

Half-warrior pose

9. Start standing on your knees, hip width apart, and then take a big step forward with the right foot, keeping your left knee on the ground. Square your hips forward and place your hands on your right thigh.

As you exhale, sink your hips forward and down. Be sure to keep approximately a 90-degree angle at the knee of your forward leg. As you inhale, return to the starting position. Repeat two more times and then stay for four to six breaths.

Bring your left forward, kneel on the other knee, and repeat on the other side.

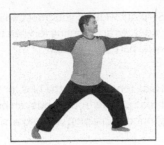

Warrior II

10. Standing in a wide stance, sideways on your mat, turn your left foot out 90 degrees and your right foot 45 degrees. An imaginary line drawn from your left heel toward your right foot should bisect the arch of your right foot.

Face forward and, as you inhale, raise your arms out to the sides parallel to the floor. As you exhale, bend your left knee over your left ankle so that your shin is perpendicular to the floor and bring your gaze over your left finger. Straighten your left leg as you inhale.

Repeat this movement two more times and then hold the bend, bringing your gaze over your right fingers. Stay for four to six breaths.

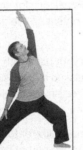

Reverse warrior

11. Still holding your warrior II pose, as you exhale drop your right hand to your back leg while at the same time reaching to the ceiling with your left hand.

Keep the bend in your front leg as you stay in this position for four to six breaths.

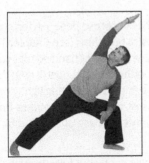

Extended side angle

12. From the reverse warrior pose, you are now going to shift your torso in the opposite direction.

On an exhalation, bring your left arm all the way to your left knee, bending the arm and resting it on the knee. At the same time, bring the right arm up and overhead (along the side of your ear), reaching forward.

Hold this position for four to six breaths and then repeat the last three poses (warrior II, reverse warrior, and extended side angle— on the other side.

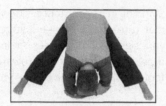

Wide stance standing twist

13. Step out wide on your mat and make sure your toes are pointing forward toward the wide part of your mat.

Hang forward from the hips for six to eight breaths. *Note:* Your hands can be on the ground or clasping your elbows.

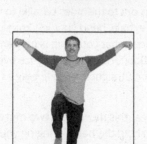

Karate kid pose

14. Standing on your mat, raise your arms out to the sides as you inhale, bringing them parallel to your shoulders (modified T-shape). Focus on a stationary spot in front of you.

As you exhale, bend your right knee, raising it toward your chest. Keep your left leg straight.

Stay in this balance for six to eight breaths and then repeat on the other side.

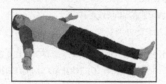

Corpse pose

15. Lie flat on your back, with your arms stretched out and relaxed by your sides, palms up (or whatever feels most comfortable).

Place a small pillow or folded blanket under your head and another large one under your knees for added comfort. Bend your knees if it feels better on your back.

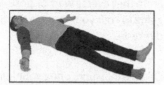

Corpse with alternate nostril breathing

16. While in corpse pose, perform alternate nostril breathing (see Chapter TK), where you place your right hand so that your thumb is blocking the right nostril (and the pinky and ring fingers are resting lightly on the left nostril, the index and middle fingers tucked against the base of the thumb).

Inhale gently but fully through the open nostril. Now, open the blocked nostril, close the other nostril, and then exhale. Inhale through that same nostril and exhale through the opposite nostril.

Repeat for 8 to 12 breaths. For more information on alternate nostril breathing, see Chapter 3.

Routine 3

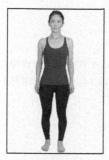

Mountain pose (with chest-to-belly breathing).

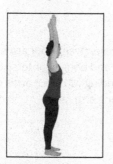

Rejuvenation sequence

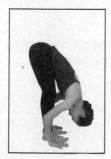

Rejuvenation sequence

1. Stand tall but relaxed with your feet at hip width; hang your arms at your sides, palms turned toward your legs. Visualize a vertical line connecting your ear, your shoulder, and the sides of your hip, knee, and ankle.

   While in this pose, employ the chest-to-belly breathing technique described in Chapter 3, taking six to eight breaths.

2. Stand in the mountain posture with your feet at hip width and arms at your sides. As you inhale, slowly raise your arms out from the sides and up overhead.

   As you exhale, bend forward from your hips and bring your head toward your knees and your hands forward and down toward the floor in the standing forward bend.

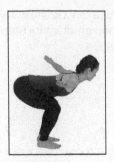

Rejuvenation
sequence

Bend your knees quite a bit and as you inhale, sweep your arms out from the sides, but only come halfway up with your arms in a T (half forward bend) and your back parallel to the floor.

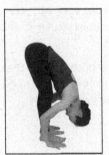

Rejuvenation
sequence

As you exhale, fold all the way down again and hang your arms in the standing forward bend.

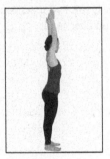

Rejuvenation
sequence

As you inhale, sweep your arms from the sides like wings and bring your torso all the way up again, standing with your arms overhead in the standing arm raise.

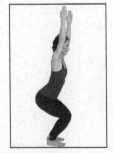

Rejuvenation
sequence

As you exhale, bend your knees and squat halfway to the floor.

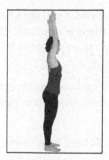

Rejuvenation
sequence

As you inhale, bring your torso all the way up again, standing with your arms overhead in the standing arm raise.

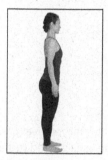

Rejuvenation
sequence

As you exhale, bring your arms back to your sides as in Step 1.

Repeat this sequence four to six times.

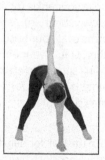

Standing twist

3. Step out wide on your mat with your toes pointing forward. As you inhale, bring your arms into a T (parallel to the floor) and lengthen your spine. As you exhale, bend forward from your hips and bring your left hand to the floor and your right arm and your head up as high as it feels comfortable.

Soften or bend your knees if you're stiff or feel any discomfort in your lower back. Remember, in Yoga, you may hold a pose, but never hold your breath.

As you inhale, return to the starting position. Repeat this movement on the same side and, on the third time, hold your left hand down and your right hand reaching up. Your head can be looking up, in the middle, or down. Stay for four to six breaths. If you want to make it more challenging, move your left hand (that's on the ground) closer to your right foot.

After holding for four to six breaths, repeat the same sequence on the other side.

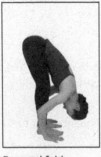

Forward fold

4. Bring your feet back to hip width and fold forward. Release your arms and hands toward the floor. Let your head hang down (to release the top of your spine).

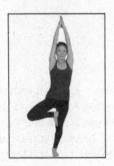

Tree pose

5. Stand upright, with your feet parallel at hip width. As you exhale, bend your right knee and place the sole of your right foot, toes pointing down, on the inside of your left leg below your knee and above your ankle (or above your knee and below your groin). As you inhale, bring your arms over your head and join your palms together. Soften your arms and focus on a nonmoving spot six to eight feet in front of you. Stay in this position for six to eight breaths. Switch sides.

REMEMBER

It's okay to use the wall for help with your balance or to have it close by just in case.

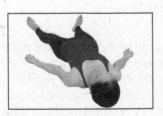

Corpse pose

6. Lie flat on your back, with your arms stretched out and relaxed by your sides, palms up (or whatever feels most comfortable).

Place a small pillow or folded blanket under your head and another large one under your knees for added comfort. Bend your knees if it feels better on your back. Stay for four to six breaths.

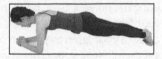

Forearm plank

7. Facing your mat, place your forearms parallel on the floor (either with palms flat or bring your palms together with interlaced fingers) and extend your legs behind you. Lift your hips as you support yourself only on your forearms and toes. Don't lift up too high; you want a flat line from your back all the way down to your legs.

If this position proves too challenging or causes any kind of pain, drop your knees to the floor for added support.

Try staying in this position for six to eight breaths, eventually working your way up to 30 breaths.

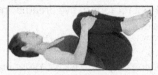

Knees to chest

8. Lie on your back and bend your knees in toward your chest. Hold your shins just below the knees. If you have any knee problems, hold underneath your thighs instead.

If you prefer, you can push back into a child's pose before flipping on to your back. (See Chapter 4 if you need to be reminded of what child's pose looks like.)

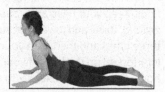

Cobra pose

9. Lie on your belly with your thumbs near your armpits, fingers forward and head down. As you inhale, pull forward and up, like a turtle coming out of a shell. Keep your buttocks relaxed. Repeat six to eight times. *Note:* While it may take some concentration, keeping your buttocks relaxed will help restore the natural (lumbar) curve in your low back.

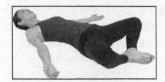

Reclined bound angle

10. Lying flat on your back, bring the soles of your feet together. (Your heels should be as close to your groin as you can comfortably get them.) Keep your arms at your sides with palms down.

Stay in this pose for six to eight breaths.

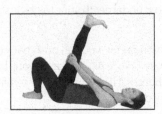

Hip opener (variation 1)

11. Begin with on your back, with your knees bent and both feet on the ground. Place your left ankle on top of your right knee. Slide your left hand through the opening and surround the back of your right thigh with both hands and pull back to your comfort level.

Hold for four to five breaths and then switch sides.

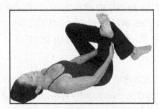

Hamstring stretch

12. Lying on your back with your legs straight, place your arms along your sides with your palms down. Bend just your left knee and put that foot on the floor. As you exhale, bring your right leg up, knee as straight as possible.

As you inhale, return your right leg to the floor. Keep your head and your hips on the ground. Raise and lower that straight leg three times and then, with your hands interlocked on the back of your right thigh, hold your leg in place for six to eight breaths.

Repeat on the other side.

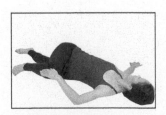

Reclined bent leg twist

13. Lie on your back with your knees bent and your feet on the ground. Bring your arms out into a T with the palms down. Hang your right thigh over your left thigh.

As you exhale, drop both bent knees to the right. As you inhale, bring them both up. Repeat three times and on the third time, stay down for six to eight breaths. Repeat on the other side by reversing thighs and the direction you drop your knees.

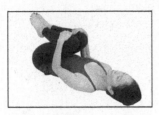

Knees to chest

14. Lie on your back and slowly bring your knees in toward your chest to tolerance. If you have knee problems, you can hold under your thighs. Stay for four to five breaths.

Note: In this pose, feel free to rock from side to side to massage your lower back.

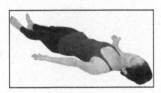

Corpse pose

15. Lie on your back with your knees bent or straight, feet on the ground, and palms up. Breathe in and out through the nose 12 to 14 times. Try to be in the moment, sensing your body, breath, and mind.

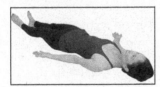

Corpse with breath work

16. Staying in corpse pose, perform the bellows variation breathing exercise described in Chapter 3. Try to do 15 to 20 breaths.

Chapter **21**

Thirty-Minute Routines for Home

I f you have a half-hour to practice, this chapter gives you three routine options. I gave this sequence a lot of consideration, oftentimes using postures to both compensate for a pose that occurred before and prepare your body for a posture that's coming up.

In each pose, I provide you with the steps to get into the pose, but I also point you to other places in this book that talk about a certain pose.

It may at first take you additional time to complete the sequence as you read the instructions next to each pose. You'll go much faster once you learn how to get into each pose.

If a particular pose seems too challenging or causes pain, modify it in a way that works for you or skip it entirely. Knowing what's good for your body and what isn't is truly a sign of being an advanced Yoga practitioner.

Routine 1

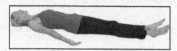

Corpse pose

1. Lie flat on your back, with your arms stretched out and relaxed by your sides, palms up (or whatever feels most comfortable). Place a small pillow or folded blanket under your head and another large one under your knees for added comfort. Bend your knees if it feels better on your back. Stay for six to eight breaths.

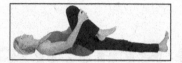

Knee to chest

2. Lie on your back with both legs straight. As you exhale, draw one knee into your chest and hold on with both hands, just below the knee cap. Bring your toes back toward you. Stay for six to eight breaths. (Keep the other leg straight, or place your foot on the ground with your knee bent if it feels better on your back.)

Note: If you're having knee problems, you can use both hands to hold underneath the knee.

Repeat on the other side.

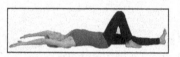

Bent leg arm raise

3. Lie on your back with one leg bent and one leg straight. Start with your arms at your side, palms down. As you inhale, bring both arms overhead. As you exhale, bring your arms back to your sides. Repeat two more times.

Next, on an inhalation, bring both arms overhead again but this time keep your arms overhead as you exhale and then inhale, trying to stretch your arms even further. On your next exhalation, bring your arms back down.

Repeat. Do the same sequence on the other side.

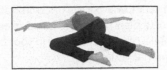

Windshield wiper

4. Lie on your back, both knees bent and feet on the ground, wide apart. Your arms are at your sides, palms down. As you exhale, drop both knees to the right. As you inhale, bring both knees back up. As you exhale, let both knees fall to the left.

Repeat three times on each side and then stay on the right for four to five breaths. Repeat, leaving your knees down on the other side.

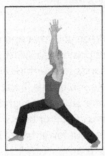

Knees to chest

5. Lie on your back and bend your knees in toward your chest. Hold your shins just below the knees. If you have any knee problems, hold the backs of your thighs instead.

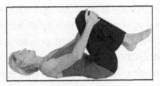

Warrior I

6. Start standing with your feet comfortably apart. As you exhale, step forward approximately 3 to 3.5 feet (or the length of one leg) with your right foot. Your left foot turns out naturally, but if you need more stability, turn it out more so that your toes point to the left.

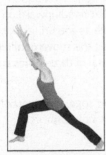

Warrior variation 1

7. Place your hands on the top of your hips and square the front of your pelvis; release your hands and hang your arms. Bend your forward knee. If you can't see your toes, step out further. Then, straighten your front leg and hang your arms.

As you inhale, raise your arms forward and overhead and bend your right knee to a right angle (so that the knee is directly over the ankle and the thigh is parallel to the floor).

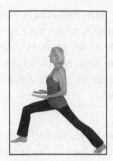

Warrior variation

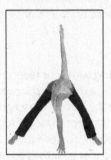

Wide stance
standing twist

If your lower back is uncomfortable, lean the torso slightly over the forward leg until you feel a release of tension in your back (see warrior variation 1).

As you exhale, return to the starting place; soften your arms, and face your palms toward each other, looking straight ahead. Repeat three times and then stay for six to eight breaths.

Bring your arms down, parallel to the floor, and pull your elbows back while extending your hands forward (palms up). As you pull your shoulder blades closer together, it may help to imagine you're holding a tray (see warrior variation 2). Stay for four to six breaths and repeat on the other side.

8. Step out wide on your mat and make sure your toes are pointing forward. As you inhale, bring your hands to your hips and lengthen your spine. As you exhale, bend from your hips, draw your stomach in, and fold forward. (Keep your knees soft or bent if you feel any discomfort in your lower back.) Place your hands on the mat.

Moving your right hand underneath your face, reach your left hand upward on your next inhale. Exhale as you bring your arm back down. Repeat this movement (on the same side) for a total of three times and then hold.

Remember: In Yoga, you may hold a pose, but never hold your breath.

If you want to make it more challenging, you can move your right hand, which is on the ground, closer to your left foot.

Repeat on the other side.

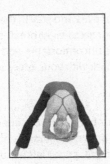

Wide stance
forward fold

9. Still folding forward, come back to the middle, bringing your hands to the floor for support, or maybe clasping your elbows.

Stay for four to six breaths.

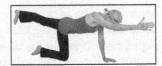

Balancing cat

10. Beginning on your hands and knees, position your hands directly under your shoulders with your palms down, your fingers spread on the floor, and your knees directly under your hips. Straighten your arms, but don't lock your elbows.

As you exhale, slide your right hand forward and your left leg back, keeping your left hand and your left toes on the floor. As you inhale, raise your right arm and left leg to a comfortable height.

Hold for four to six breaths; repeat on the other side.

To challenge yourself, you can move the extended arm and leg side-to-side slowly.

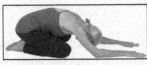

Child's pose

11. Starting on your hands and knees, place your knees about hip width apart with your hands, just below your shoulders. You want your elbows straight but not locked.

As you exhale, sit back on your heels; rest your torso on your thighs and your forehead on the floor. You don't have to sit all the way back. Reach your arms forward with your palms down or lay your arms back on the floor beside your torso with your palms up (or forward with your palms on the floor).

Close your eyes and stay in the folded position for six to eight breaths. (If this position is uncomfortable, you can always lie on your back with your knees into your chest.)

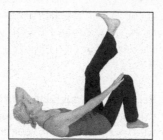

Slide ups

12. Lie on your back with your knees bent and your feet flat on the floor. Bend your left elbow and place your left hand on the back of your head just behind your left ear.

Raise the left leg as close to vertical (90 degrees) as possible, but keep your knee slightly bent. Draw the top of your foot toward your shin to flex your ankle and place your right palm on your right thigh near your pelvis. As you exhale, sit up slowly halfway and slide your right hand toward your knee.

Keep your left elbow back in line with your shoulder and look at the ceiling. Don't throw your head forward.

Repeat this movement four more times and then switch to the other side. (If you want extra support for your neck, use both hands behind your head.)

If you want to make it more challenging, stay up for an extra breath before coming back down.

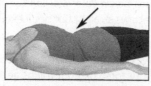

Locks

13. Lie on your back with your legs straight (or knees bent with feet on the ground if more comfortable). Exhale completely and then tighten your anal sphincter, pull your abdomen inward, and hold for five counts. Release. Take a normal inhale and repeat. Try to do eight to ten rounds.

For a more detailed description of the locks see Chapter 18.

If you have heart issues or high blood pressure, talk with your doctor to see whether this routine is appropriate for you.

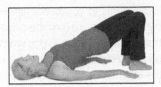

Bridge pose

14. Lie on your back with your knees bent, feet flat on the floor at hip width, and your arms at your sides with palms turned down. As you inhale, raise your hips to a comfortable height As you exhale, return your hips to the floor.

Repeat four to eight times.

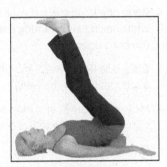

Supported half shoulder

15. Choose a foam block, bolster, or several folded blankets, and place them near you. Lie on your back with your knees bent and your feet flat on the floor at hip width, resting your arms along the sides of your body with your palms down. As you inhale, raise your hips and then insert the prop of your choice under the top of your hips or sacrum.

Note: As an option you can simply sit sideways at a wall and then swing both legs up, lie back, and rest your hands at your sides.

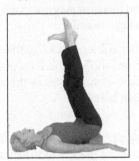

Point and flex feet

Slowly bring both legs straight up and then back toward your head so that you're in a V-shape looking up at your feet. Rest your hands at your sides, palms down. If your legs are straight, your knees should not be locked. Simply relax in the posture. Let your breath be smooth on both the inhalation and exhalation.

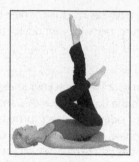

One leg bent

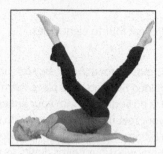

Scissor the legs

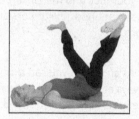

Leg split

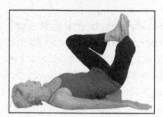

Bound angle

Stay for two to three minutes, gradually working up to five minutes.

You have the options to add the following movements as you become more comfortable in the posture (see the photographs, though some of these you won't be able to do if you choose to simply put your legs up the wall):

- Point and flex your feet

- Rotate your ankles

- Bend one knee toward your hip and point while flexing and rotating the other foot (do both sides)

- Bring one leg forward and one leg back in a scissors (not at the wall)

- Move three times and then stay open on each side for three to five breaths

- Open your legs into a split

- Move your legs in and out three times and then just stay out in the split for five to eight breaths

- Bring the legs back together, bend at the knees, and join the soles of your feet together supported by the wall for five to eight breaths

Finally, bring your legs up one last time and just breathe until it's time for you to come out.

When you come down, slowly bend and lower your legs until they touch the floor. Pull your prop out, lower your legs, and just relax.

REMEMBER

When you're ready to sit up, don't lead by lifting your head forward. Roll to one side and then press up to prevent neck strain.

WARNING

While you should always talk with your doctor before starting any kind of a Yoga program, inverted postures like this one should be avoided if you are pregnant or have any of the following conditions:

- High blood pressure
- Hiatal hernia
- GERD
- Retinopathy
- First few days of your menstrual cycle

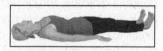

Corpse pose

16. Go into the corpse pose, which is the same resting position you were in when you started this sequence (Step 1). Stay for six to eight breaths.

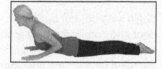

Cobra

17. Lie on your belly with your thumbs near your armpits, fingers forward and head down. As you inhale, pull forward and up, like a turtle coming out of a shell. Keep your buttocks relaxed. Repeat six to eight times.

Note: You may choose to use the modified cobra pose in this step.

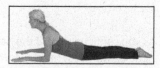

Modified cobra

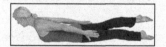

Locust variation

18. Lie on your belly with your legs spread at hip width and the tops of your feet on the floor; extend your arms back along the sides of your torso with your palms on the floor and rest your forehead on your mat face down.

As you inhale, raise your chest and one leg (arms can stay on the ground). Exhale as you lower back down. Repeat three times and hold for three to five breaths.

Keep your eyes forward so that you won't bring your head too far backward.

Repeat on the other side.

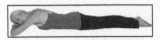

Prone corpse pose

19. Because you're already on your stomach, place your hands underneath your forehead, feet wider than hip width apart, and just rest for six to eight easy breaths.

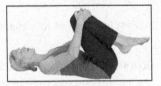

Knees to chest

20. Because the previous two poses were back bends, your body probably feels like it wants to fold, which moves your spine in the opposite direction. You can actually start out in child's pose or move right into knees-to-chest. Both poses compensate for the backward bending and give you a chance to rest.

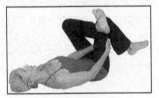

Hip opener (variation 1)

21. Begin lying on your back, with your knees bent and both feet on the ground. Place your left ankle on top of your right knee. Slide your left hand through the opening, surround the back of your right thigh with both hands, and pull back to your comfort level.

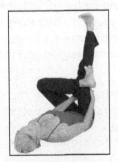

Hip opener (variation 2)

22. As you continue to hold the back of your right leg with both hands, slowly straighten the right leg three times and then just hold it straight for four to five breaths.

Repeat Steps 22 and 23 on the other side.

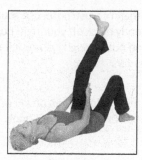

Hamstring stretch

23. Lying on your back with your legs straight, place your arms along your sides with your palms down. Bend just your right knee and put that foot on the floor. As you exhale, bring your left leg up, knee as straight as possible.

As you inhale, return your left leg to the floor. Keep your head and your hips on the ground. Raise and lower that straight leg three times and then, with your hands interlocked on the back of your thigh, hold your leg in place for six to eight breaths.

Repeat on the other side.

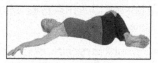

Reclined bent leg twist

24. Lie on you back with your knees bent and your feet on the ground. Bring your arms out into a T with the palms down.

As you exhale, drop both bent knees to the left. As you inhale, bring them both up. Repeat three times and on the third time, stay down for six to eight breaths. Repeat on the other side.

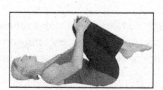

Knees to chest

25. Lie on your back and slowly bring your knees in toward your chest to tolerance. If you have knee problems, you can hold under your thighs. Stay for six to eight breaths.

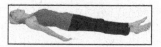

Corpse pose

26. Lie on your back with your knees bent or straight, feet on the ground, and palms up. Breathe in and out through the nose, 8 to 12 times. Try to be in the moment, linking your body, breath, and mind.

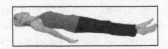

Corpse with left nostril breathing

27. Staying in corpse pose, use your right thumb to gently block off your right nostril. Breathe in and out through just the left nostril for 12 to 15 breaths.

For more information on left nostril breathing, see Chapter 3 in this book.

Routine 2

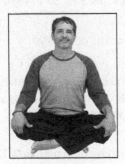

Easy pose

1. Sit on your mat with your legs straight out in front of you; place your hands on the floor beside your hips with your palms down and fingers pointing forward. Shake your legs up and down a few times to get the kinks out.

Bend your knees and cross your ankles in front of you, sitting comfortably.

Rest your hands on your knees with your arms relaxed and palms down. Lengthen your spine by stretching your back in an upward motion, balance your head over your torso, and look straight ahead. Take six to eight breaths.

Note: To help you sit straighter and lessen the strain on your back, try sitting on a bolster or stack of blankets for all seated poses.

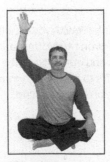

Arm raises

2. While in a comfortable seated position (stay in easy pose), raise your right arm over head on an inhalation; lower your arm on the exhalation.

Raise your left arm on your next inhalation; lower your arm on the exhalation.

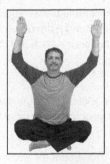

Raise both arms overhead on your next inhalation; lower both arms on the exhalation.

Repeat this sequence one time.

3. Still in your seated position (easy pose), take a big inhale. As you exhale, put both hands in front of you on your mat (palms down) and slide out as far as your body wants to go. Inhale back up.

Repeat two more times and hold the stretch forward for four to six breaths.

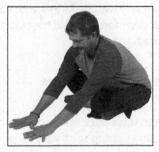

Seated cross-legged forward bend

4. Continue sitting comfortably in a cross-legged position. Place your left palm on the floor, near your left hip.

As you inhale, raise your right arm out to the side and up above your head beside your left ear. As you exhale, slide your left hand across the floor out to the left, letting your torso, head, and right arm follow as you bend to the left.

Note: Don't let your buttocks come off the floor as you bend.

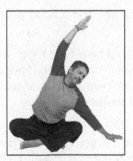

Seated side bend

Inhale back to the upright position. Repeat two more times and hold the stretch for three to five breaths.

Repeat on the other side.

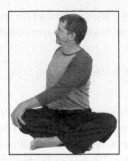

Seated twist

5. Still in a comfortable cross-legged position, place your left hand palm down on top of your right knee. Put your right hand down behind your right hip.

As you inhale, extend your spine upward. As you exhale, twist your torso and head to the right.

Repeat this movement for two more breaths, gradually twisting farther with each exhalation, but don't force it. Hold the twist for six to eight breaths.

Repeat on the other side.

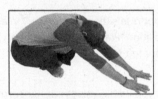

Seated cross-legged forward bend

6. From this seated position, try sliding forward again — just to see if your range of motion has increased.

Hold the stretch for four to six breaths.

Get on your hands and knees, with your wrists under your shoulders and knees under your hips. Your head and back should be in a neutral position.

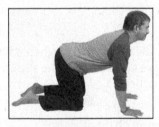

Cow pose

7. Inhale as you drop your belly toward the mat and raise your chin upward. (This is cow pose.)

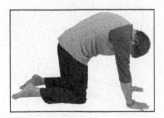

Cat pose

8. As you exhale, draw your chest inward and round your back upward. You are now looking downward, bringing your chin toward your chest. (This is cat pose.)

Repeat this movement two more times.

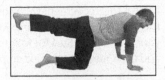

Cat-cow variation

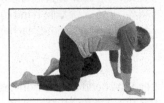

9. Still on your hands and knees, bring your chin toward the ceiling as you inhale, at the same time lifting and extending your left leg out behind you. As you exhale, bring your leg and bent knee in as your back comes into the cat posture described in the previous step.

Repeat this movement two more times and then switch to the other side.

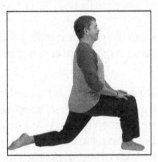

Half-warrior pose

10. Start standing on your knees, hip width apart, and then take a big step forward with the right foot, keeping your left knee on the ground. Square your hips forward and place your hands on your right thigh.

As you exhale, sink your hips forward and down. Be sure to keep approximately a 90-degree angle with the knee of your forward leg.

As you inhale, return to the starting position. Repeat two more times and then stay for four to six breaths.

Repeat these steps on the other side.

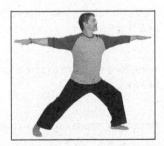

Warrior II

11. Standing in a wide stance, sideways on your mat, turn your left foot out 90 degrees and your left foot 45 degrees. An imaginary line drawn from your left heel toward your right foot should point to the center of the arch of your right foot.

Face forward and, as you inhale, raise your arms out to the sides parallel to you're the floor. As you exhale, bend your left knee over your left ankle so that your shin is perpendicular to the floor Straighten your left leg as you inhale.

Repeat this movement two more times and then hold the bend, bringing your gaze over your left fingers. Stay for four to six breaths and then move to the next step.

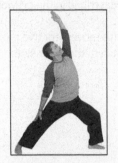

Reverse warrior

12. Still holding your Warrior II pose, as you exhale drop your right hand to your back leg while at the same time reaching to the ceiling with your left hand.

Keep the bend in your front leg as you stay in this position for four to six breaths.

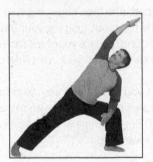

Extended side angle

13. From the reverse warrior pose, shift your torso in the opposite direction.

On an exhalation, bring your left arm all the way to your left knee, bending the arm and resting it on the knee. At the same time, bring the right arm up and overhead (along the side of your ear), reaching forward.

Hold this position for four to six breaths and then repeat this sequence of last three poses (warrior II, reverse warrior, and extended side angle) on the other side.

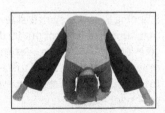

Wide stance forward

14. Step out wide on your mat with your toes pointing forward.

Hang forward from the hips for six to eight breaths.

Note: Your hands can be on the ground or clasping your elbows.

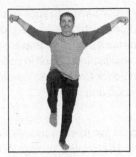

Karate kid pose

15. Standing on your mat, raise your arms out to the sides as you inhale, bringing them parallel to your shoulders (modified T-shape). Focus on a stationary spot in front of you.

As you exhale, bend your right knee, raising it toward your chest. Keep your left leg straight.

Stay in this balance for six to eight breaths and then repeat on the other side.

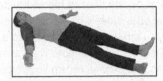

Corpse pose

16. Lie flat on your back, with your arms stretched out and relaxed by your sides, palms up (or whatever feels most comfortable). Place a small pillow or folded blanket under your head and another large one under your knees for added comfort. Bend your knees if it feels better on your back. Stay for six to eight breaths.

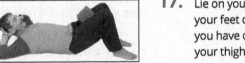

Yoga crunches with a block

17. Lie on your back with your knees bent and your feet on the floor. Place a foam block (if you have one) or folded blanket between your thighs, close to your groin.

Place your thumbs behind your earlobes pressing against your jaw bone. Spread your fingers behind the back of your head. Keep your elbows wide.

As you exhale, squeeze the block or blanket, tilt the front of your pelvis toward your navel, and with your hips on the ground, slowly lift your head and chest as you sit up halfway.

Keep your elbows wide and your gaze toward the ceiling. Don't pull your chin to your chest. Repeat eight to ten times.

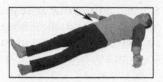

Yoga locks

18. Lie on your back with your legs straight (or knees bent with feet on the ground, if more comfortable). Exhale completely, tighten your anal sphincter, pull in your abdomen, and hold for five counts. Take a normal inhalation and repeat.

Try to do five to eight rounds. For a more detailed description of Yoga locks, see Chapter 18.

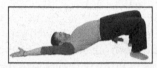

Bridge pose

19. Lie on your back with your knees bent, feet flat on the floor at hip width, and your arms at your sides with palms turned down. As you inhale, raise your hips to a comfortable height and raise your right arm overhead. As you exhale, return your hips and arm to the floor.

As you inhale again, raise your hips to a comfortable height and raise your left arm overhead. On your exhalation, lower your hips and arm back to the floor.

On your next inhalation, raise your hips to a comfortable height and both arms overhead. As you exhale, return your hips and arms to the floor.

Repeat this sequence three to four more times.

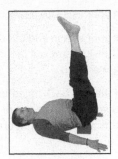

Supported half shoulder

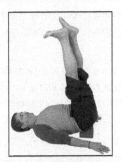

Point and flex feet

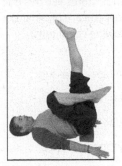

One leg bent

20. Choose a foam block, bolster, or several folded blanket, and place them near you. Lie on your back with your knees bent and your feet flat on the floor at hip width, resting your arms along the sides of your body with your palms down. As you inhale, raise your hips up and then insert the prop of your choice under the top of your hips or sacrum.

TIP

As an option, you can simply sit sideways at a wall and then swing both legs up, lie back, and rest your hands at your sides.

Slowly bring both legs straight up and then back toward your head so that you're in a V-shape looking up at your feet. Rest your hands at your sides, palms down. If your legs are straight, your knees should not be locked. Simply relax in the posture. Let your breath be smooth on both the inhalation and exhalation.

Stay for two to three minutes, gradually working up to five minutes.

You have the options to add the following movements as you become more comfortable in the posture (see the photographs, though you won't be able to do some of these if you choose to simply put your legs up the wall):

- Point and flex your feet

- Rotate your ankles

- Bend one knee toward your hip and point while flexing and rotating the other foot (do both sides)

- Bring one leg forward and one leg back in a scissors (not at the wall)

- Move three times and then stay open on each side for three to five breaths

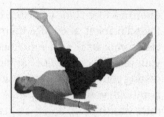
Scissor the legs

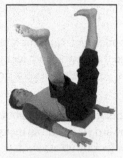
Leg split

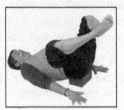
Bound angle

- Open your legs into a split

- Move your legs in and out three times and then just stay out in the split for five to eight breaths

- Bring the legs back together, bend at the knees, and join the soles of your feet together for five to eight breaths

Finally, bring your legs up one last time and just breathe until it's time for you to come out.

When you come down, slowly bend and lower your legs until they touch the floor. Pull your prop out, lower your legs, and just relax.

REMEMBER

When you're ready to sit up, don't lead by lifting your head forward. Roll to one side and then press up to prevent neck strain.

Note: While you should always talk with your doctor before starting any Yoga program, inverted postures like this one should be avoided if you are pregnant or have any of the following conditions:

- High blood pressure

- Hiatal hernia

- GERD

- Retinopathy

- First few days of menstruation

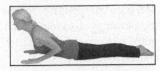

Cobra

21. Lie on your belly with your thumbs near your armpits, fingers forward, and head down. As you inhale, pull forward and up, like a turtle coming out of a shell. Keep your buttocks loose. Repeat six to eight times.

Note: While it may take some concentration, keeping your buttocks loose will help restore the natural (lumbar) curve in your low back.

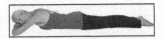

Reverse corpse pose

22. Stay on your belly and just rest for six to eight breaths. Turn your head to either side or place your hands under your forehead and feet wider than hip width apart. Stay for six to eight breaths.

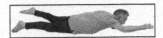

Half locust

23. Stay on your belly with your legs separated at hip width and the tops of your feet on the floor; extend your right arms in front of you with your palm down and your forehead resting on your mat. Note: If this posture seems too challenging at the moment, just do a second set of the cobra pose (#21). As you inhale, raise your chest, the right arm and left leg. Exhale as you lower back down. Repeat three times and hold in the lifted position for three to five breaths. Repeat on the other side.

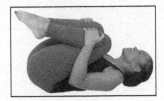

Knees to chest

24. Lie on your back and bend your knees in toward your chest. Hold your shins just below the knees. If you have any knee problems, hold underneath your thighs instead.

This pose compensates for the back bending (by allowing you to fold, which is the opposite of the two previous poses) and gives you a chance to rest.

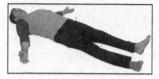

Corpse with alternate nostril breathing

25. While in corpse pose, perform four-part breathing

Repeat for 8 to 12 breaths.

For more information on four-part breathing, see Chapter 3 in this book.

Routine 3

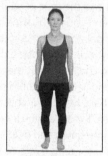

Mountain pose (with chest-to-belly breathing)

1. Stand tall but relaxed with your feet at hip width; hang your arms at your sides, palms turned toward your legs. Visualize a vertical line connecting your ear, your shoulder, and the sides of your hip, knee, and ankle.

While in this pose, employ the chest-to-belly breathing technique described in Chapter 3, taking six to eight breaths.

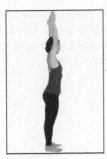

Rejuvenation
sequence

2. Stand in the mountain posture with your feet at hip width and arms at your sides. As you inhale, slowly raise your arms out from the sides and up overhead.

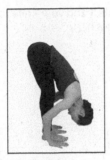

Rejuvenation
sequence

As you exhale, bend forward from your hips and bring your head toward your knees and your hands forward and down toward the floor in the standing forward bend.

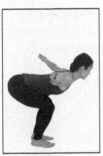

Rejuvenation
sequence

Bend your knees quite a bit and as you inhale, sweep your arms out from the sides, but only come halfway up with your arms in a T (half forward bend) and your back parallel to the floor.

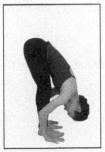

Rejuvenation
sequence

As you exhale, fold all the way down again and hang your arms in the standing forward bend.

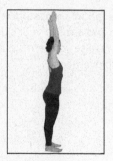

Rejuvenation
sequence

As you inhale, sweep your arms from the sides like wings and bring your torso all the way up again, standing with your arms overhead in the standing arm raise.

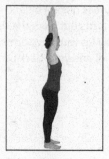

Rejuvenation
sequence

As you exhale, bend your knees and squat halfway to the floor.

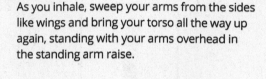

Rejuvenation
sequence

As you inhale, bring your torso all the way up again, standing with your arms overhead in the standing arm raise.

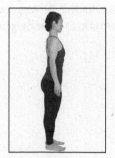

Rejuvenation
sequence

As you exhale, bring your arms back to your sides as in Step 1.

Repeat this sequence four to five times.

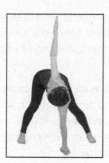

Standing twist

3. Step out wide on your mat and make sure that your toes are pointing forward. As you inhale, bring your arms into a T (parallel to the floor) and lengthen your spine. As you exhale, bend forward from your hips, bring your left hand to the floor, and lift your right arm and your head up as high as it feels comfortable.

   Soften or bend your knees if you're stiff or feel any discomfort in your lower back.

REMEMBER

In Yoga, you may hold a pose, but never hold your breath.

As you inhale, return to the starting position. Repeat this movement on the same side and, on the third time, hold your left hand down and your right hand reaching up. Your head can be looking up, in the middle, or down. Stay for four to six breaths.

If you want to make it more challenging, move your left hand, which is on the ground, closer to your right foot.

After holding for four to six breaths, repeat the same sequence on the other side.

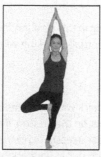

Tree pose

4. As you exhale, bend your right knee and place the sole of your right foot, toes pointing down, on the inside of your left leg between your knee and your ankle (or between your knee and your groin). As you inhale, bring your arms over your head and join your palms together. Soften your arms and focus on a nonmoving spot six to eight feet in front of you. Stay in this position for six to eight breaths. Switch sides.

   And it's okay to use the wall for help with your balance or to have it close by just in case.

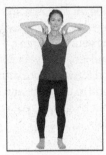

Bent arm shoulder rolls

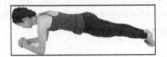

Corpse pose

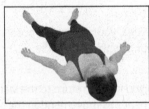

Forearm plank

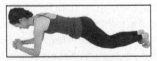

Modified forearm plank

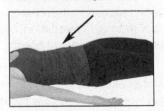

Yoga locks

5. Standing upright, extend both arms outward, palms up. Now bend your elbows and bring your fingertips to the top of each shoulder.

Making circles with your elbows, allow your shoulders to move up, back, and down. Go in one direction three to four times and then reverse the circles in the opposite direction for three to four times.

6. Lie flat on your back, with your arms stretched out and relaxed by your sides, palms up (or whatever feels most comfortable). Place a small pillow or folded blanket under your head and another large one under your knees for added comfort. Bend your knees if it feels better on your back. Stay for six to eight breaths.

7. Facing your mat, place your forearms parallel on the floor (either with palms flat or bring your palms together with interlaced fingers) and extend your legs behind you. Lift your hips as you support yourself only on your forearms and toes. Don't lift up too high; you want a flat line from your back, all the way down to your legs.

If this position proves too challenging or causes any kind of pain, drop your knees to the floor for added support.

Trying staying in this position for six to eight breaths, eventually working your way up to 30 breaths.

8. Lie on your back with your legs straight or knees bent with feet on the ground, if more comfortable. Exhale completely, tighten your anal sphincter, and pull in your abdomen and hold for five counts. Take a normal inhale and repeat.

Try to do five to eight rounds.

For a more detailed description of Yoga locks, see Chapter 18.

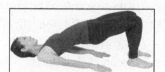

Bridge pose

9. Lie on your back with your knees bent, feet flat on the floor at hip width, and your arms at your sides with palms turned down. As you inhale, raise your hips and right arm to a comfortable height. (Try to touch the floor with the back of your right hand.) As you exhale, return your hips to the floor.

Repeat four to six times.

Choose a foam block, bolster, or several folded blankets, and place them near you. Lie on your back with your knees bent and your feet flat on the floor at hip width, resting your arms along the sides of your body with your palms down. As you inhale, raise your hips and then insert the prop of your choice under the top of your hips or sacrum.

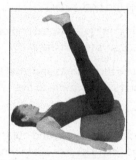

Supported half-shoulder

Note: As an option you can simply sit sideways at a wall and then swing both legs up, lie back, and rest your hands at your sides.

Slowly bring both legs straight up and then back toward your head so that you're in a V-shape looking up at your feet. Rest your hands at your sides, palms down. If your legs are straight, your knees should not be locked. Simply relax in the posture. Let your breath be smooth on both the inhalation and exhalation.

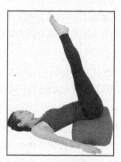

Point and flex feet

Stay for two to three minutes, gradually working up to five minutes.

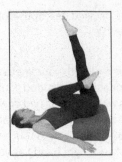

One leg bent

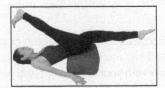

Scissor the legs

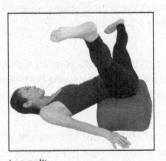

Leg split

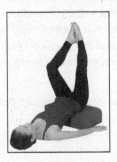

You have the options to add the following movements as you become more comfortable in the posture (see the photographs, though some of these you won't be able to do if you choose to simply put your legs up the wall):

- Point and flex your feet

- Rotate your ankles

- Bend one knee toward your hip and point while flexing and rotating the other foot (do both sides)

- Bring one leg forward and one leg back in a scissors (not at the wall)

- Move three times and then stay open on each side for three to five breaths

- Open your legs into a split

- Move your legs in and out three times and then just stay out in the split for five to eight breaths

- Bring the legs back together, bend at the knees, and join the soles of your feet together for five to eight breaths

Finally, bring your legs up one last time and just breathe until it's time for you to come out.

When you come down, slowly bend and lower your legs until they touch the floor. Pull your prop out, lower your legs, and just relax. When you're ready to sit up, don't lead by lifting your head forward. Roll to one side and then press up to prevent neck strain.

10. While you should always talk with your doctor before starting any Yoga program, inverted postures like this one should be avoided if you are pregnant or have any of the following:

- High blood pressure
- Hiatal hernia
- GERD
- Retinopathy
- First few days of menstruation

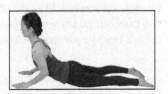

Corpse pose

11. Once again, return to this resting pose to allow your body to fully recover from the inversion for six to eight breaths.

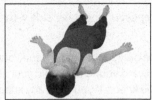

Cobra pose

12. Lie on your belly with your thumbs near your armpits, fingers forward and head down. As you inhale, pull forward and up, like a turtle coming out of a shell. Keep your buttocks relaxed. Repeat six to eight times.

Note: While it may take some concentration, keeping your buttocks relaxed will help restore the natural (lumbar) curve in your low back.

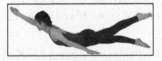

Locust variation

13. Lie on your belly with your legs separated at hip width and the tops of your feet on the floor; extend your arms in front of you with your palms down and your forehead resting on your mat.

Note: If this posture seems too challenging at the moment, just do a second set of the cobra pose (Step 12).

As you inhale, raise your chest and one leg. You could also raise the opposite arm. Exhale as you lower back down. Repeat three times and hold in the lifted position for three to five breaths.

WARNING

As you lift your chest, be careful not to pull your head up and back too far (to the point of pain).

Repeat on the other side with opposite pairs.

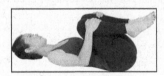

Knees to chest

14. Lie on your back and bend your knees in toward your chest. Hold your shins just below the knees. If you have any knee problems, hold underneath your thighs instead.

This pose compensates for the back bending by allowing you to fold — the opposite of the two previous poses and gives you a chance to rest. Hold for six to eight breaths.

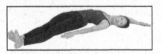

Banana pose

15. Lie on your back with your legs straight and resting on the mat. (Your shoulders are on the mat as well.) Bring your right arm overhead, with your left arm at your side. Keeping your hips on the mat, slide both legs sideways, to the left.

The C-shaped curve your body is now making resembles a banana shape.

Hold this lateral bend for six to eight breaths and then switch to the other side.

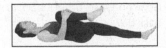

Knee to chest

16. Lie on your back with both legs straight. As you exhale, draw one knee into your chest and bring your toes back toward you. Stay for six to eight breaths. Keep the other leg straight or place your foot on the ground with your knee bent if it feels better on your back.

Repeat on the other side.

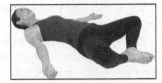

Reclined bound angle pose

17. Lying flat on your back, bring the soles of your feet together. (Your heels should be as close to your groin as you can comfortably get them.) Keep your arms at your sides with palms up.

Stay in this pose for six to eight breaths.

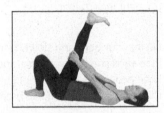

Hamstring stretch

18. Lie on your back with your knees bent and feet on the ground at hip width. Place your arms at your sides with your palms down.

Straighten your right leg and let it rest on the mat. Keep your head and your hips on the ground. As you exhale, raise the straight leg and as you inhale lower the leg three times. Then, with your hands interlocked on the back of your thigh, hold your leg in place for three to four breaths.

Then, shift the right leg out about six inches to the right and pull it gently backward. Hold for three to four breaths.

Then, bring it back to center and shift it inward about six inches. Pull it gently backward again. Hold for three to four breaths (be careful when you move inward since this can be more sensitive than the other positions).

Gently release, bring it back to center and back down.

Repeat on the other side.

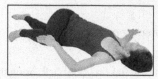
Reclined bent leg twist

19. Lie on your back with your right knee held against your chest. (The left leg should be straight if it feels okay on your back.) Bring your arms out into a T with the palms down. As you exhale, use your left hand to guide your right knee across your body to the left, into a twist. Inhale the knee back up to midline and drop it again (to the left) on your exhalation. After moving down and up three times, hold the twist for four to five breaths.

Repeat on the other side with the left knee up, right leg straight.

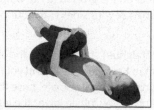
Knees to chest

20. Lie on your back and slowly bring your knees in toward your chest to tolerance. If you have knee problems, you can hold under your thighs. Stay for four to five breaths.

Note: In this pose, feel free to rock from side to side in order to massage your lower back.

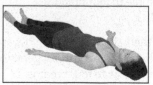
Corpse pose

21. Lie on your back with your knees bent or straight, feet on the ground, and palms up. Breathe in and out through the nose, six to eight times. Try to be in the moment, linking your body, breath, and mind.

22. Staying in corpse pose, perform the bellows variation breathing exercise described in Chapter 3. Try doing 12 to 15 breaths.

6

The Part of Tens

Chapter **22**

Ten Tips for Your Yoga Practice: On the Mat

There's a dangerous way of looking at Yoga that says every posture must conform to a traditional view of the pose. I work hard in this book to give you an alternative perspective — in fact, an opposite point of view. If Yoga is going to serve you, it must fit you.

The challenge, of course, is that everyone is different — bodies are different and need different things. That's why I can't share with you a one-size-fits-all solution. Without a doubt, the best way to shape your Yoga practice is to listen to what your body needs. Of course, a skilled Yoga teacher may intuitively know what Yoga practices will best serve you and help you discover them. Yet a teacher can only make an educated guess; only you can truly know.

The following list represents what I think are the most critical takeaways from this book, relating specifically to your physical Yoga practice.

Avoid Pain at All Cost

Yoga shouldn't hurt. Not ever! Yet sometimes even teachers who try to keep you safe may not make the right call. That's because they're not actually in your body — but you are.

WARNING

Don't let your ego draw you into doing anything that causes you pain or even serious discomfort. The "No pain, no gain" adage has no place in Yoga.

See Chapter 1 for more on avoiding injury and an overactive ego.

It's Okay to Change Your Mind

Sometimes, you don't know if something is bad or good for you until you try it. In Yoga, you may think that a certain posture or movement may be beneficial — maybe it will stretch you out or make you stronger. Sometimes, however, you don't know what hurts until you give it a try. And that's perfectly okay — as long as you've given yourself permission to change your mind. Always feel free to back off if that's what your body's telling you to do.

Modify when Necessary

The concept of modification may be the most important lesson I can teach you. You can easily see that your body is not the same now as it was when you were 20 years old. I also want it to be easy for you to accept that fact. As your body changes, so, too, should your Yoga practice. You won't need to modify everything, but definitely modify when you need to.

Chapter 4 identifies common modifications to Yoga's most popular poses.

Choose Forgiving Limbs

This tip is actually part of my "modify when necessary" advice. Yet it is such an important concept — particularly for the 50-plus yogi — that I'm identifying it as a separate tip, all on its own.

Clearly, one of the best ways you can modify a posture is by allowing your arms or legs (or, more precisely, your elbows and knees) to bend. While this modification may take you further away from the traditional form of the pose, it may ultimately bring you closer to what's beneficial about the pose in the first place.

See Chapter 1 for more on forgiving limbs.

REMEMBER

Function takes precedent over form (at least, for my students and me).

Prepare the Muscles and Joints

Moving in and out of poses before holding them is a great way to warm up the joints and muscles — a process used by many athletes, and even more important to do as you get older. Also, in my discussion of Proprioceptive Neuromuscular Facilitation in Chapter 1, I refer to a principle that says tensing a muscle before you relax it will make it lengthen further. Moving in and out of poses before you hold them may have a similar effect.

Use the Power of Your Breath

If maintaining a slow breath rate helps to keep your blood pressure and heart rate low and reduces stress and anxiety, then it is critically important for you to believe that the process of breathing is just as important as the pose itself. Pay attention to your breath; let it be part of your practice. (For more on breathing, see Chapter 3.)

Selecting a Studio

Yoga studios are everywhere today. And, while it is great to have a lot of convenient options, it's also challenging to find just the right class at just the right studio. This challenge is particularly true when so many public classes are clearly targeted for younger people who want to build cardio into their Yoga sessions or focus on traditional poses. If you decide a public class is the way to go, take the time to investigate. Make sure the teacher of a particular class is eager to focus on your particular needs.

For more on selecting a studio, see Chapter 1.

Assessing Yoga Online

Yoga videos (like the ones found on YouTube) are just as pervasive as the studios themselves. And, once again, so many of them are geared to the younger Yogi, where a very traditional expression of a pose is the ultimate target.

Take the time to preview a particular video and make sure it is appropriate for you. If you take the time to dig deep, you can find videos that will keep you safe.

Chapter 1 talks more about videos online.

Be Realistic about Your Time

The problem with overestimating how much time you're going to give to a Yoga practice is that if you fall short, it's easy to convince yourself that you have somehow failed. Of course, that's just not true. Most people have busy lives, and some days can be busier than others. That's why I include 5-minute, 15-minute, and 30-minute routines in Chapters 19, 20, and 21, respectively.

REMEMBER

Even if your day is so full you only have time for 5 minutes, see that as a victory. A little bit is better than nothing at all.

Include Meditation

While Western medicine is slow to confirm many of the Yoga principles that many in the field take for granted, an abundance of studies highlight the various benefits of a regular meditation practice. The conclusions of those studies often have very positive implications for the 50-plus population — specifically as it relates to brain structure and cognitive performance. (See Chapter 5 for more on the power of meditation.) Each day, when you go to your mat, make meditation part of your routine.

IN THIS CHAPTER

» **Thinking good things**

» **Eating good things (and probably not as much)**

» **Finding a cardio workout**

» **Developing a meditation routine**

» **Creating a community**

Chapter **23**

Ten Tips for Your Yoga Practice: Off the Mat

Anyone who thinks that Yoga is just about poses, about being especially mobile or flexible, is really ignoring what some people would argue is the most important part of the practice. Yoga is a philosophy of life — and, as such, offers a lot of important insights on ways to find more joy in life and reduce suffering.

Of course, you can get a multitude of health benefits from a regular practice, but just as many off-the-mat practices can enrich your life and relationships in many important ways.

While Chapter 22 focuses primarily on some important takeaways relating to your physical practice, in this chapter, I discuss all the other areas of insight Yoga has to offer.

Take Your Vitamin G

Because there is a direct link between the mind and the body — between what you think and how you physically feel — finding a place of gratitude will bring that positive energy right from your thoughts into your cells.

In Chapter 8, I talk about creating a gratitude journal where you can record, on a daily basis, the things for which you're most grateful. I believe gratitude is a powerful practice and so I put it at the top of my off-the-mat tips.

Eat Well

Your Yoga teacher, and often times even your doctor, may not have the specialized training to adequately assess your diet. Yet what and how much you eat is certainly related to your overall health. While Yoga traditionally suggests you probably need to eat less as you get older, exactly what your diet should look like must be determined by a true expert. (For more about seeing a nutritionist or other health professional, see Chapter 6.)

REMEMBER

If there's one thing that Yoga teaches, it's that we are all individuals, with individual needs. Instead of a Yoga teacher telling you to not eat this or eat more of that, considering letting a health professional be your guide.

Find a Cardio Workout You Like

Clearly, certain types of Yoga are more physically demanding than others and probably get your heart rate up more, such as a physical flow practice or a typical power Yoga class. But if you're not in those sessions, it's important to get your heart rate up, to exercise your heart muscles, so consider another type of cardio exercise, like walking, swimming, or biking. In most cases, Yoga is going to have the opposite effect by bringing your heart rate down. (See Chapter 6 for more about the importance of finding a cardio routine.)

Get a Good Night's Sleep

Getting the proper amount of sleep is critical. You should address any sleeping issues you have and explore the tools that Yoga has to offer that may help. Sometimes a Yoga routine itself will help make you tired. Or, you may also choose to try a routine like the Yoga Sleep at Home routine that I include in Chapter 8, which employs the concept of Yoga sleep or *Yoga Nidra*. If you don't get enough sleep, it may be hard to meditate because you might keep nodding off during your practice.

Avoid the Blue Light before Bedtime

The original Yoga masters did not, of course, talk about blue light. But if they were living today, I'm sure they would. Blue light is a problem stemming from modern technology — from all electronic devices with screens — and it needs to be mentioned in a Yoga context because it works directly against the Yoga tools that fight insomnia or stress. You should cut down on the amount of time you're exposing yourself to blue light or block it with special glasses or an app. And especially avoid using your electronic devices (even TV) before trying to sleep. (See Chapter 8 for more about the problem with blue light.)

Communicate to Enhance Intimacy

Some Yoga masters would argue that one of the goals of Yoga philosophy, in general, is to help improve personal relationships. As you come to know yourself better through Yoga, you can in turn be more empathetic and understanding of the people around you. That can be especially true with a life partner. Sharing your thoughts, desires, and fears can be extremely challenging. But such candor can break down walls and make what's good even better. (See Chapter 8 for more on using Yoga to build intimacy.)

Find Time to Meditate Off the Mat

Developing some kind of meditation is so important that I want to encourage you to develop a routine separate from your physical Yoga practice — off the mat, if you will. Maybe you're going to find the time while sitting at your desk, walking the beach, sitting on the couch, or lying in bed. Try some different techniques and different locations. See what works. (For more about meditation, see Chapter 5.)

Say Goodbye to Your Ego

Your ego can create a competition in your mind with the person on a nearby mat. Or even if you do Yoga alone, sometimes you try to prove something to yourself. In both of these cases, when you want to show how flexible you are, Yoga can ultimately lead to injury — and this is the danger of listening to your ego instead of your body. One of the benefits of being older is that we sometimes find it easier to let go of ego-driven concepts and expectations. (See Chapter 1 for more on this topic.)

Invite Others to Join In

I try to avoid using a lot of Sanskrit or Yoga jargon in this book, but I can't help mentioning the term *sangha*. Basically, it's a term that means *community*, and I want to encourage you to bring people into your Yoga world or join people who are already there. There's a lot of power to be found in connecting with others, and Yoga can be a means of achieving that. Even if it's just doing Yoga together.

Start Today

You may have heard the saying, "If I knew I was going to live this long, I'd have taken better care of myself." Well, it's never too late, so start now.

And if it's true that your body often reflects what's going on in your mind, make sure there's something good to draw upon — something celebratory.

Index

B

backbends, anterior hip replacements and, 189

balance
about, 125–126
alignment poses, 128–133
poses for, 128–133
proprioception, 126
tips for poses, 127–128
Yoga for, 11

Balancing Cat pose
about, 97, 128–129
for bone health, 205
in 15-minute routines, 265
for lower back pain, 144, 145
in 30-minute routines, 285

ball-and-socket joints, 178

Banana pose, 310

bandhas, 246

bee breath, 44–45

"Bee Breath to Get Anxiety to Buzz Off" (McCall), 44–45

bellows variation routine
in 30-minute routines, 312
about, 42

belly breathing, 40, 153, 163–164

belly lock, 246, 247–248

bending
legs, 215–216
from the waist, 197–199

benefits
of balanced diets, 86–88
of breathing exercises, 36
of meditation, 71–73
of stress reduction, 110
of Yoga, 7–13
of Yoga for knees, 166–167

Bent Arm Shoulder Rolls pose
in 30-minute routines, 306
for upper back, 158–159

Bent Leg Arm Raise pose
about, 141–142
in 15-minute routines, 262
in 5-minute routines, 252
in 30-minute routines, 282

Bent Leg Supine Twist pose
about, 55–56
for lower back pain, 146–147

Bhavanani, Ananda Balayogi (doctor), 40

blankets, 27–28

blocks, 25–27

blood flow, reversing, 69

blue light, 111–112, 321

blue-light-filtering glasses, 111–112

Boat pose
about, 56
for knees, 170–171

bodies
listening to your, 50
Yoga benefits for, 10–12

body scan, 115–118

bolsters, 28–29

bone density, 196

bone health, routine for, 199–210

bone spurs, 211

bone strength. *See* osteoporosis

Bound Angle pose
anterior hip replacements and, 189
in 15-minute routines, 278
for hamstrings, 180, 181, 186
for hips, 180, 181, 186
for hormonal changes, 234

breathing
about, 35
advanced approaches to, 40–45
alternate nostril
in 15-minute routines, 272–273
in 30-minute routines, 302
about, 43–44

approaches to, 39–45

for arthritis, 227, 228

balance and, 128

bee breath, 44–45

bellows variation routine, 42, 312

belly, 40, 153, 163–164

benefits of exercises in, 36

Chest-to-belly

about, 40

for bone health, 199–200

in 5-minute routines, 256

cooling breath, 231–233

diaphragmatic, 152–153

extending exhalations, 37–38

focus

about, 39, 89

for upper back, 154

four-part, 38, 39

importance of, 317

left nostril

about, 42–43

in 15-minute routines, 267

in 5-minute routines, 253

in 30-minute routines, 292

leveraging, 36–39

nasal, 36–37

for neck, 152–153

relationship with movement, 38–39

Seated Belly Breathing, 163–164

through your nose, 36–37

for upper back, 152–153

Yoga for improved, 10

Bridge pose

about, 31, 32, 57

for hormonal changes, 237, 238

for knees, 173–174

in 30-minute routines, 287, 298, 307

C

calcium, 197

cardio, 88, 320

Cat pose

about, 95–96

for arthritis, 217–218, 223–224

in 15-minute routines, 270

in 30-minute routines, 294–295

causes

of arthritis, 212

of extension faults, 138

of flexion faults, 137

of menopause, 230

of pelvic floor issues, 245–246

Chair pose, 174

Chair Twist pose, 93–94

cheat sheet (website), 3

Chest-to-belly breathing

about, 40

for bone health, 199–200

in 5-minute routines, 256

Child's pose

about, 57–58

anterior hip replacements and, 189

in 15-minute routines, 265

for hormonal changes, 236–237

posterior hip replacements and, 190

in 30-minute routines, 285–286

chin lock, 246

chronic asthma, 149, 152. *See also* upper back

chronic conditions, Yoga for, 12

Chronic Obstructive Pulmonary Disease (COPD), 152

circadian rhythm, 111

classes, selecting, 14–17

clothing, 24–25

Cobra pose

about, 58, 137, 139

in 15-minute routines, 266, 277

in 30-minute routines, 289, 301, 309

community centers, classes at, 17

competitive nature, 53–54

cooling breath, 231–233

COPD (Chronic Obstructive Pulmonary Disease), 152

About the Author

Larry Payne, Ph.D., C-IAYT, E-RYT500, is an internationally respected Yoga teacher, author, and a founding father of Yoga therapy in America. Dr. Payne cofounded the International Association of Yoga Therapists, now in 50 countries, and the Yoga curriculum at the UCLA School of Medicine. He is also the founder of the Yoga Therapy Rx and Prime of Life Yoga certification programs at Loyola Marymount University, the corporate Yoga program at the J. Paul Getty Museum, and the original Back Program at the Rancho La Puerta Fitness Spa.

In 2000, he was the first Yoga teacher to be invited to The World Economic Forum in Davos, Switzerland and, in 1996, he performed the first documented headstand at the North Pole! He founded Samata International Yoga and Health Center in Los Angeles 1980, where he continues to teach groups and individuals.

Dr. Payne is coauthor of the international bestseller *Yoga For Dummies* (John Wiley & Sons, Inc.), *Yoga Basics* (John Wiley & Sons, Inc.), *Yoga Rx* (Broadway Books), *The Business of Teaching Yoga* (Samata International), and *Yoga Therapy and Integrative Medicine* (Basic Health Publications, Inc). He is featured in the *Prime of Life Yoga and Yoga Therapy Rx* DVD series (available at Samata.com) and most recently appears globally online at *Yoga International*, *Glo*, and *Yoga Download*. His website is *Samata.com*.

Dedication

I dedicate this book to the love of my life, Merry Aronson, and to my beloved family: my mother, Dolly; my father, Harry, in heaven; Harold; Chris; Lisa; Sasi; Maria; and Natale.

And to my students, who are my greatest teachers.

Author's Acknowledgments

First and foremost, I am grateful for the amazing contributions of my editor, Don Henry, without whom this book would not have been possible. Also, many thanks to Don for his wonderful photography and videography. Enormous gratitude also goes to our official Yoga expert, Dr. Matthew J. Taylor, PT, PhD, C-IAYT, and my other health professional friends and colleagues who contributed their expertise to our Yoga Therapy chapters: Dr. Ananda Balayogi Bhavanani; Richard Miller, PhD; Shannon Collins, PT, CMPT; Lori Rubenstein Fazzio DPT, PT, C-IAYT; Shelly Prosko, PT, CPI, C-IAYT; and Andrew Yun, M.D. Much appreciation to my first Yoga teachers: TKV Desikachar and family, Indra Devi, AG Mohan and family, Swami Vishnu Devananda and Raghavan Dass; and to my board of advisors comprised of Rick Morris, D.C.; Richard Usatine, M.D.; David Allen, M.D.; Art Brownstein, M.D.; LeRoy R. Perry, D.C.; David Boyer, M.D; MarK K. Urman, M.D.; Steve Paredes, D.C.; Mark J. Kelly, M.D.; Professor Zhou-Yi Qiu, Fancy Fechser, Amanda Charney, Sir Sidney Djanogly, and Steve Ostrow.

Great big thanks to Tracy Boggier at Wiley for believing in this project and presenting it to Wiley and AARP. Kelly Ewing is our great senior editor at Wiley and helped make the whole process a pleasure. At AARP, thanks to Jodi Lipson, Director of AARP Books, and Lorrie Lynch, Director of Features Content, who helped to shape this book for the 50-plus audience.

Also much appreciation to our great Yoga models: Yonetta Asin, Marynn Blanchard, Deanna Courtney, Judy Ellis, Guy Gabriel, Lisa Henry, De Jur Jones, Monique Johnson, Joe Lopez, Greg Miguel, Martha Orgado, Pamela Rosenthal, Peter Smyth, and Sachie K. Yoshitake. Makeup: Taria Groce.

And, always, to Merry Aronson, whose love, support, and expertise make everything better.

Publisher's Acknowledgments

Senior Acquisitions Editor: Tracy Boggier

Project Editor: Kelly Ewing

Technical Editor: Matthew J. Taylor, Ph.D.

Proofreader: Debbye Butler

Production Editor: Siddique Shaik

Photographer: Don Henry

Cover Image: © adamkaz/Getty Images